DATE DUE

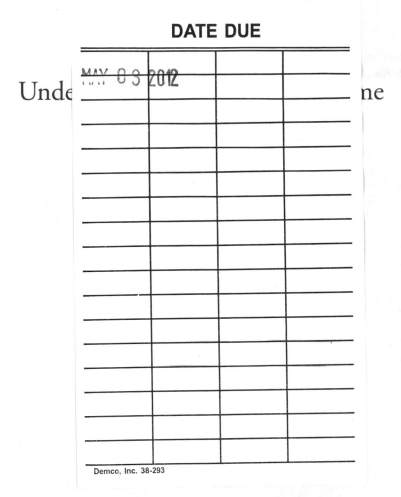

Unde

MAY 0 3 2012

ne

Demco, Inc. 38-293

Understanding Fragile X Syndrome

A Guide for Families and Professionals

Isabel Fernández Carvajal
and David Aldridge

Jessica Kingsley *Publishers*
London and Philadelphia

Epigraph from García Márquez 1967 on p.5 is reproduced by
permission of Agencia Literaria Carmen Balcells.
Table 4.1 from Hagerman et al. 2008 on p.50 is reproduced by permission of Randi Hagerman.

First published in 2011
by Jessica Kingsley Publishers
116 Pentonville Road
London N1 9JB, UK
and
400 Market Street, Suite 400
Philadelphia, PA 19106, USA

www.jkp.com

Library of Congress Cataloging in Publication Data
Fern?ndez Carvajal, Isabel.
  Understanding fragile X syndrome : a guide for families and professionals /
Isabel Fern?ndez Carvajal and David Aldridge.
      p. ; cm. -- (JKP essentials)
  Includes bibliographical references and index.
  ISBN 978-1-84310-991-4 (alk. paper)
  1. Fragile X syndrome. I. Aldridge, David, 1947- II. Title. III. Series:
JKP essentials.
  [DNLM: 1. Fragile X Syndrome. 2. Ataxia--genetics. 3. Tremor--genetics.
QS 677]
  RJ506.F73F47 2011
  616.85'884--dc22

                                   2010046069

British Library Cataloguing in Publication Data
A CIP catalogue record for this book is available from the British Library

ISBN 978 1 84310 991 4

Printed and bound in Great Britain

To the memory of Antonio

'There is always something left to love'

Gabriel García Márquez
One Hundred Years of Solitude
London: Jonathan Cape, 1967

CONTENTS

List of Figures, Tables and Boxes

Figures

Tables

Boxes

Chapter 1

WHAT IS FRAGILE X SYNDROME?

When Samuel is born he is a lovely baby boy. When he is eight months old his parents become worried because he doesn't seem to be developing as they expect. Something does not appear to be quite right about their baby. He has difficulty in sitting unsupported and then he is not able to crawl. His development milestones, like walking, do not appear as in other children of a similar age. The family doctor tells the parents, 'Do not worry, some children develop later. Just be patient.' The parents are patient but still retain their suspicions that something is wrong with their child. Eventually Samuel begins to walk, but by the age of two years his parents are concerned that he is not talking. Again, the family doctor tells them not to worry as language often comes later.

Eventually Samuel does speak a few words, like 'Mama' and 'Papa', and can echo words that are said to him. By the time he is four years old and ready for infant school, his developmental delay becomes clear. In contrast to his peers, his communicative abilities are limited and Samuel's teacher has difficulties in integrating Samuel in the classroom because he is constantly active. Samuel has difficulty maintaining the attention he needs to learn in the classroom and to relate to his classroom peers. His teacher calls his parents and tells them of her concerns about his language difficulties and his relational problems. She says that it is difficult to teach Samuel because of his limited attention and constant activity. This is when Samuel is referred to a specialist, in this case a neuro-paediatrician.

The neuro-paediatrician diagnoses that Samuel has an autism spectrum disorder and prescribes medication for controlling Samuel's hyperactivity.

Meanwhile, Samuel has a new baby brother, Julian. Samuel's condition does not improve. He has psychological problems in school and it becomes clear that other children are bullying him because of his disabilities. On referral to a child psychologist, his parents are told that the problems are a result of Samuel being jealous of his new baby brother.

When Samuel is six years old, the family seek further help in the nearest large city from a specialist in child intellectual disability. Reviewing Samuel's appearance, developmental history and behaviour, including his school difficulties, the specialist decides to carry out a genetic test. The results of the test show that Samuel has Fragile X syndrome.

On the basis of this test, the doctor asks if there are other siblings. As we have seen, Samuel's baby brother Julian is now part of the family, and the parents have the same concerns about him that they had about Samuel. Julian does not appear to be developing as they expect and the doctor decides to carry out the genetic test. Julian proves also to have Fragile X syndrome. The parents had no idea beforehand that this was a problem in their respective families.

The child specialist then sends the parents to a genetic counsellor as they need to be aware of their own genetic status before they decide whether to have further children. The counsellor will ask them about their own families of origin and previous problems of developmental delay – even medical problems that their grandparents have. If the parents had known earlier that a second child could be affected by Fragile X syndrome, their decision to have the child might have been affected.

As the reader will see, the genetic problem of Fragile X can be tested quite easily. The ramifications for Samuel, Julian, their parents and the rest of the family, however, are complex. These are not medical decisions alone but serious ethical, familial and social decisions, which include informed decision-making about family planning knowing that there is a possibility of disability for any subsequent children.

BACKGROUND

Fragile X syndrome is the most common form of inherited developmental disability even though is often under-diagnosed. The syndrome is caused by a change in the genetic make-up itself, as we will see in Chapter 2. It was known formerly as Martin-Bell syndrome, named after the physician, James Purdon Martin, and the geneticist, Julia Bell, who first discovered it in 1943. Although we have known about the syndrome for over 60 years, there is still a limited awareness of the problem, even amongst health care practitioners, as it affects both children and adults.

Fragile X is found in all races and at all socio-economic levels. Recent statistics indicate that 1 in 2500–4000 males and 1 in 4000–6000 females are affected, and that approximately 1 in 260 females and 1 in 300–800 males are carriers of a gene pre-mutation.

The syndrome usually manifests itself as problems in the acquisition of language and a delay in the child's development. The degree of intellectual disability in Fragile X syndrome varies from borderline to severe in affected individuals.

Intellectual disability appears in children under the age of 18 and many parents will have suspected that something is not quite right with their child's development before early schooling is contemplated. Intellectual disability is recognised as having an intellectual level below 70–75 points as measured by standard intelligence tests, and the presence of limitations in daily living skills. These skills include the ability to produce and understand language. Academic skills such as reading, writing and arithmetic are also challenged, and this may mean specialised schooling should be considered. The everyday skills needed for living at home, the self-care skills needed for daily hygiene and staying healthy, and the social skills of living in the community may also be under-developed. All these skills are necessary for beginning early schooling. However, some forms of mild developmental disability are only recognised when the child first starts school. There is a general problem in that parents often recognise that their child is not moving or communicating as expected at an earlier age than health care professionals will acknowledge, which means a delay in diagnosis.

Intellectual disability is a condition which has an impact on individuals and families in various ways and degrees of severity. Fragile X syndrome can be passed on by individuals in a family from one generation to the next, even if those family members in the older generation have no apparent signs of their genetic condition. In some families a newly diagnosed individual may be the first family member to exhibit symptoms, and this can have consequences for the rest of the family. While the initiator for recognising the syndrome is a genetic disorder expressed by the individual, the consequences for a family are behavioural, emotional, intellectual, relational and social. The individual child may be considered to be developmentally delayed, yet the whole family experiences the consequences of that delay.

Fragile X syndrome is expressed as a range of symptoms from intellectual and learning disabilities to more severe cognitive or intellectual disabilities, all encompassed by the term 'developmental delay'. Symptoms can include characteristic physical and behavioural features with variable degrees of severity. These features may include hyperactivity. A Fragile X disorder is also one of the known contributors to 'autistic-like' behaviours or autism spectrum disorders. Although not all children with Fragile X syndrome will have an autism spectrum disorder, approximately one third of all children diagnosed with Fragile X syndrome also have some degree of autism.

Initially, concerns about Fragile X were with the genetic disorder and its consequences for children and the status of their developmental delay. Nowadays, we know that there are other Fragile X-associated syndromes, including Fragile X-associated tremor/ataxia syndrome (FXTAS), which is a condition that affects balance, tremor and memory in some older pre-mutated carriers, and Fragile X-associated Primary Ovarian Insufficiency (FXPOI), in some pre-mutated carrier women. The latter is a problem with ovarian function that can lead to infertility and early menopause.

Because of its variable clinical presentation, diagnosis of Fragile X syndrome is not possible on a clinical basis alone, and the condition has to be considered in the differential diagnosis of any child presenting with learning disabilities, developmental delay, mental retardation, autistic features or hyperactivity. It is thought that a great number of people affected by Fragile X worldwide have not been correctly diagnosed.

Confirmation of the diagnosis necessitates genetic analysis. Diagnosis of Fragile X is achieved through DNA tests, and genetic counselling is available in many countries for information and support. Although there is currently no cure for Fragile X, drugs therapies which may improve attention impairment and hyperactivity are available. Early intervention with other therapies, including speech, physical, psychological and music therapies, all provide real benefit to people with the syndrome.

In this book, we will attempt to show a broad picture from the gene to the family level. It is important to remember that while there have been major advances in genetics that allow us to recognise the changes that take place in genetic structure, the consequences of these changes are extremely complex. While we have excellent medical, psychological, social and educational resources, bringing those resources together is a challenge. Informed parents can be the instigators and coordinators of these resources, challenging professionals to meet their needs. There is a growing trend towards translational medicine. Translational medicine is an approach where natural scientists, like molecular biologists, pharmacologists and geneticists, are encouraged to 'translate' their findings into language that clinicians can understand or carry out research that is directly relevant to clinicians' needs. Similarly, clinicians are being encouraged to 'translate' their own research ideas into projects that can be investigated by natural scientists. This is often called the 'bench' to 'bedside' approach. We suggest that this approach is taken a step further and that researchers and clinicians also include the families and their knowledge bases because, ultimately, it is the families for whom this knowledge is gleaned and they who bear the consequences of genetic change.

Chapter 2

UNDERSTANDING HEREDITY

Genetic Factors and Inheritance

Almost every human disease has a genetic component. Genes, behaviour and the environment interact and influence the course of disease and health. It makes sense then to understand what happens in this interaction in order to develop potential means of treating genetic problems. Even if no treatments currently exist, we can discover how we may ameliorate the impact of hereditary conditions through counselling, behavioural therapies and modifying and improving environmental conditions.

GENES AND CHROMOSOMES

Fragile X syndrome is *not* a disease that is caught through an infection; it is a condition that is inherited, and changes can occur from one generation to the next. Because the intergenerational change can be an expansion (or a reversal), this is known as a 'dynamic mutation'. In order to understand Fragile X syndrome, it is important to understand how human genes and chromosomes influence this condition (see Figure 2.1).

In the figure we can see (a) the whole person, which contains (b) the cells with their nuclei, which contain (c) the chromosomes, which are composed of segments of (d) DNA (deoxyribonucleic acid) formed from the nucleotides adenine (A), cytosine (C), guanine (G) and thymine (T), which are combined in specific sequences.

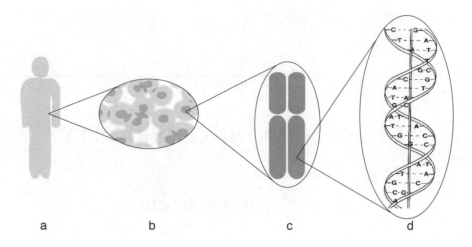

a   b   c   d

Figure 2.1 From human being to nucleotide

Every cell in the body has a set of chromosomes. There are 23 pairs of chromosomes in a human cell nucleus. Mothers and fathers contribute a chromosome to make each pair. One of these pairs is the sex chromosomes which determine whether you are male or female, plus some other body characteristics. The other 22 pairs of chromosomes determine the rest of the body's make-up (see Figure 2.2).

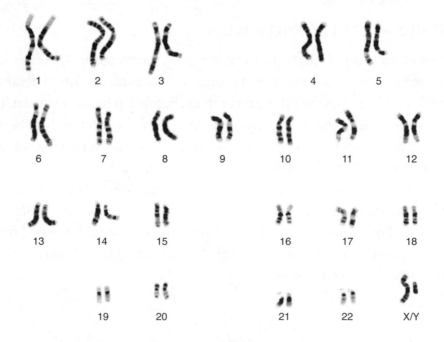

Figure 2.2 The 23 chromosome pairs including the XY chromosome pair

However, for the sex cells, or gametes, there is only a single set of 23 chromosomes. The sex chromosomes are the X chromosome and the Y chromosome, and it is these that participate in determining the sex of the person. Females have two X chromosomes in their cells. Males have both X and Y chromosomes in their cells. The egg cells, in a female, all contain an X chromosome. Sperm cells, in a male, contain either an X or a Y chromosome. It is the male, then, who determines the sex of the offspring when fertilisation occurs, by passing on either an X chromosome or a Y chromosome.

A baby boy will have only one X chromosome, which is inherited from his mother at conception, and at the same time he receives a Y chromosome from his father forming the XY chromosome pair. A baby girl will inherit two X chromosomes, one from each parent (see Figure 2.3).

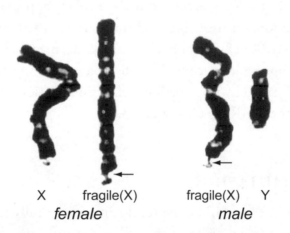

X   fragile(X)   fragile(X)   Y
female   *male*

Figure 2.3 Location of the Fragile X gene (FMR1) on the X chromosome

Each chromosome contains many genes. The gene is the basic physical unit of inheritance and contains the information needed to specify traits. Traits are specific characteristics like eye colour and height. Genes vary in size, from just a few thousand pairs of nucleotides (or 'base pairs') to over two million base pairs. Genes are segments of DNA located in chromosomes. A gene is a distinct stretch of DNA that carries the instructions for a specific function: it tells each of your cells what to do and when to do it. Humans have approximately 23,000 genes arranged on their chromosomes.

The function of most genes is to encode instructions on how to make proteins or produce other molecules that help cells assemble proteins. It is these proteins that influence how the body develops. Some proteins are very important in the developing brain where they are involved in establishing the location of nerve cells as well as the connections between those nerve cells. Proteins are made of smaller units called 'amino acids', which are attached sequentially to each other in long chains. It is the sequence of an amino acid that determines each protein's structure and its specific function. Scientific knowledge is rapidly expanding but it is still limited in that we know a lot about protein structure but are still discovering about function.

Fragile X syndrome is caused by a dynamic mutation in a gene called FMR1. This gene is located on the longer arm of the X chromosome. Fragile X takes its name from the broken appearance at the bottom of the long arm of this X chromosome, where we find the Fragile X gene (FMR1) in people with this syndrome (see Figure 2.3). This broken appearance is caused by an expansion of a small part of the sequence formed by the repetition of a trinucleotide CGG, in the beginning of the FMR1 gene at Xq27.3.

DYNAMIC MUTATION

The mutation in the FMR1 gene results in a specifically related protein, FMRP, not being made in the cell at the right time and in the correct amount. The production of this protein is blocked because the gene is switched off. The exact role of the FMRP protein in the brain is not yet known, although it is thought to regulate protein synthesis. The consequences are what we see as Fragile X syndrome.

In disorders that, like Fragile X, are caused by a trinucleotide expansion as a dynamic mutation, we find an abnormally large allele. This allele is not associated with clinical symptoms but it can expand into a full mutation when transmitted to the child, called a 'pre-mutation'. The size of change in the repeated sequence occurs from one generation to another and this is known as a 'dynamic mutation', where the gene becomes unstable. This repetition can reverse – that is, get smaller – but we are concerned here with the increase in repeats of the building blocks that eventually cause the syndrome itself. These repeats are referred to here as 'CGG repeats', which are short sequences of DNA known as a 'microsatellite'. CGG is an abbreviation of cytosine–guanine–guanine. Cytosine and guanine are nucleotides. Nucleotides are the basic building bocks of DNA. If the CGG repeats expand, in the case of Fragile X syndrome to more than 200, then the gene is effectively silenced because of its methylation with consequences for the production of the necessary FMRP protein (see Figure 2.4).

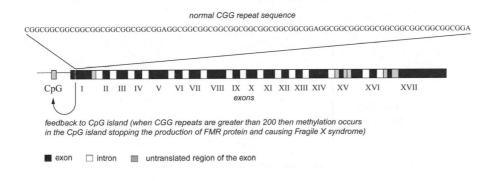

Figure 2.4 Feedback to the CpG island preventing the production of FMR protein

'Methylation' refers to a chemical process in the body that is used to turn chromosomal information off or on. In people with Fragile X syndrome, it is this process of methylation which causes the disease, turning genetic information off or 'silencing' it. Near the FMR1 gene, there is a regulatory site called a CpG island (see Figure 2.5). In most people, the site is not methylated. As a result, the cell can use the FMR1 gene for the production of Fragile X Mental Retardation Protein (FMRP). However, in people with Fragile X syndrome, the CpG island is methylated and the cell is unable to produce the protein.

The most frequent mutation of the FMR1 gene is an expansion of a small part of the sequence formed by the repetition of a trinucleotide

CGG, in the beginning of the FMR1 gene at Xq27.3, accompanied by abnormal methylation in over 98 per cent of affected individuals. This means in effect that the gene is 'turned off' or 'silenced' and therefore lacks expression. Having more than 200 CGG repeats starts methylation of the FMR1 gene in almost all cases. Methylation stops the synthesis of protein and, as we have seen, the absence of protein causes Fragile X syndrome. What we do not know is why having too many CGG repeats triggers methylation.

The stability of these CGG repeats seems to be linked to the inclusion of another nucleotide sequence, AGG. This AGG sequence occurs like a punctuation mark after every nine or ten CGG repeats. If this does not occur, then it is the probable source of the expanded sequence of CGG repeats being passed on to the next generation.

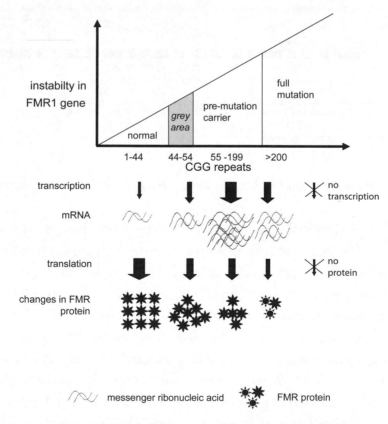

Figure 2.5 CGG allele repeats and their influence on FMRP production and the instability of the FMR1 gene

There are four allele classes according to the CGG repeat tract in the FMR1 gene:

1. *Normal or common alleles* appear in the general population; the repeat tract contains up to 40 CGG repeats, with 29 to 30 repeats being the most common.

2. *Intermediate alleles* with a range of 44 to 54 CGG repeats that are not usually associated with instability of the repeat tract.

3. *Pre-mutation carriers* with a range of 54 to 200 CGG repeats that are associated with an instabiliy of the CGG repeat. This instability means that these CGG repeats can expand to a larger pre-mutation allele or expand into the full mutation range in the next generation. Pre-mutation carriers are unmethylated, so they have FMRP protein.

4. *Full mutation*, when the number of CGG repeats is more than 200 and leads to an inactivation of the FMR1 gene, thus preventing it from synthesising the FMRP protein. We call this full mutation Fragile X syndrome (see Figure 2.5).

CONSEQUENCES

Individuals with Fragile X syndrome may have varying degrees of developmental delay, variable levels of intellectual disability, and behavioural and emotional difficulties.

Males are typically more severely affected than females. Most males have intellectual disability. Only one third to one half of females have significant intellectual disability. Fragile X can be passed on in a family by individuals who have no apparent signs of this genetic condition. In some families a number of family members appear to be affected, whereas in other families a newly diagnosed individual may be the first family member to exhibit symptoms.

Some carriers of pre-mutation in Fragile X may suffer Fragile X-associated tremor/ataxia syndrome (FXTAS), which is a condition affecting balance, tremor and memory in some older gene carriers. Female carriers may suffer Fragile X-associated Primary Ovarian Insufficiency (FXPOI), which is a problem that can lead to infertility and early menopause in some female gene carriers.

HOW IS FRAGILE X SYNDROME INHERITED?

As we mentioned above, women carry two X chromosomes in their cells but men have only one X chromosome. The male transmits his only X chromosome to all his daughters, while he transmits his Y chromosome to his male children. Therefore, all the female children of a male with pre-mutation in the gene FMR1 will be pre-mutation carriers. The extent of this pre-mutation will not be exactly that of the father, and may be slightly smaller or greater.

A female, however, has two X chromosomes and transmits one or the other with the same probability to her child. Therefore, a female with a pre-mutation has a 50 per cent risk of transferring her altered X chromosome to her male and female children. Another difference in female, compared to male carriers is that the pre-mutation tends to increase from one generation to the next, with rare exceptions (see Figure 2.6).

The full mutation causing the syndrome is always inherited from the mother, while the pre-mutation in a girl may be inherited from either mother or father. In Figure 2.7 we see how a male with pre-mutation transmits it to his daughters but not to his sons; his daughters may then transmit it as a full mutation to their offspring. If it is the female who transmits a pre-mutation, this will normally be greater in the following generation, where it could become a full mutation (more than 200 CGG repeats in a sequence).

All expansions in the range of the full mutation are always inherited from the maternal side and depend mainly on the number of CGG repeats of the pre-mutation itself. The instability of FMR1 alleles appears related to the length of the uninterrupted CGG repeat sequence. Longer repeat sequences are more likely to undergo an expansion mutation than shorter ones.

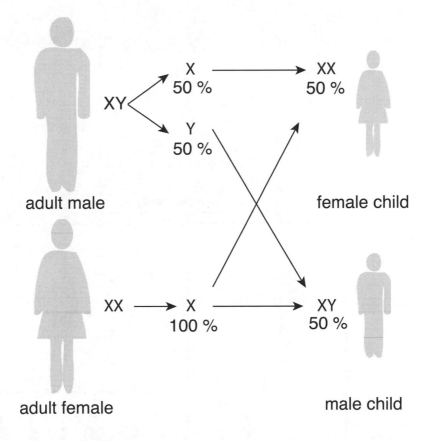

Figure 2.6 Normal patterns of inheritance of the X and Y chromosomes

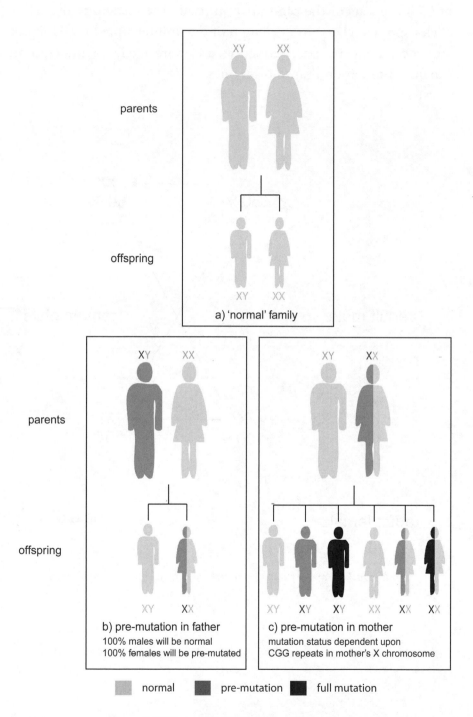

Figure 2.7 The possible combinations of inheritance
from parents with pre-mutation to offspring

Possibilities of offspring in mother with pre-mutation

As shown in Figure 2.8, a woman with a pre-mutation has the possibility, in every pregnancy, of having 'normal' sons and daughters to whom she passes on her normal X chromosome. She also risks passing on her pre-mutated X chromosome. When this happens, it can keep its pre-mutated status or expand to a full mutation in some or all of her sons and daughters.

The larger the pre-mutation in females, the more unstable it is and therefore the more probable it is that it will expand into a full mutation. On the other hand, it must be taken into account that the risk of suffering from Fragile X syndrome depends not only on inheriting the full mutation but also on the gender of the child. It is estimated that more than a half of females with a full mutation do not present clinical manifestations of Fragile X syndrome. Affected females may show a certain degree of intellectual disability that varies from borderline cases (with an IQ around 70), to moderate intellectual disability, to that of an intellectual disability equal to affected males, although a minor degree of disability is the most frequent.

Possibilities of offspring in father with pre-mutation

All of the sons of a father with a pre-mutation will inherit his Y chromosome, so they will not be at risk from his X chromosome, but he will pass his pre-mutated X chromosome to all of his daughters, who will thus have a pre-mutated X chromosome as well.

Possibilities of offspring in mother with full mutation

A mother carrying a fully mutated X chromosome has a 50 per cent chance with each pregnancy of having 'normal' sons and daughters when she passes on her normal X chromosome and a 50 per cent risk of having sons and daughters with Fragile X syndrome if she passes on her full mutated X chromosome (see Figure 2.8).

Possibilities of offspring in father with full or mosaic mutation

Fathers with a full mutation will not pass this mutation on to their sons but most likely will pass on a pre-mutation to their daughters (see Figure 2.8). It was previously thought that all males with full mutations have only pre-mutations in their sperm, but there are rare reports of daughters with full mutations born to males with full/mosaic mutations.

A small percentage of full mutation carriers have pre-mutations in a detectable proportion of their cells; they are termed 'size mosaics'. Mosaicism is a condition in which cells within the same person have a different genetic make-up. This condition can affect any type of cell, including blood cells, egg and sperm cells and skin cells. In a person with Fragile X syndrome, there may be two populations of cells with different numbers of CGG repeats (size mosaicism) within one individual. This mosaicism can have a demonstrable effect on the functionality of the gene. Males with mosaic patterns are less severely affected and they have, on average, higher IQs, presumably because they express some FMRP. However, the range of severity overlaps.

ARE ALL COMPLETE MUTATIONS ALIKE?

As we have seen earlier, in female cells there will be two X chromosomes but only one of these X chromosomes will be active in every cell. For females who carry the full mutation, the percentage of active X chromosomes with the normal repeat allele compared to the full mutation allele can modify the severity of the symptoms, as expected for any X-linked condition. On average, about one third to one half of females who carry the full mutation are significantly affected with Fragile X syndrome. Males' mosaicism status can modify their clinical and behavioural features. Predicting the severity of the symptoms of Fragile X syndrome is, therefore, difficult.

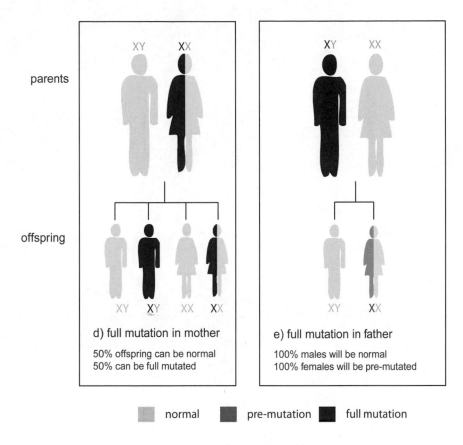

Figure 2.8 The possible combinations of inheritance from parents with full mutation to offspring

Chapter 3

THE COMMON SYMPTOMS
OF FRAGILE X SYNDROME

Fragile X syndrome is the most common inherited cause of autism and intellectual disabilities. It is expressed as a range of symptoms: intellectual and learning disabilities, and characteristic physical and behavioural features, which may include hyperactivity. It is also one of the known contributors for autistic spectrum disorders or autistic-like behaviours (gaze avoidance, repetitive behaviours, hand flapping, hand biting, touch avoidance).

Most cases of Fragile X syndrome are recognised by a clinician in contact with the child and parents together. The parents can fill in essential information about the behavioural characteristics of the child at home, or about family background regarding developmental delay or intellectual disability. There are observable clinical features that add up to the suspicion that a child has Fragile X syndrome. This can lead to a simple genetic test to establish the source of the disorder. Symptoms are usually milder in females. As we will see later, there are many clinical features and many of them are to be found in normal child behaviour.

Features include:

- developmental delay in the child being presented

- poor eye contact

- hyperactivity

- continued repetitions of words or phrases

- short attention span

- double-jointedness

- responds negatively to touch (tactile defensiveness)

- large or prominent ears

- hand flapping

- large testicles

- hand biting

- a family history of developmental delay.

CLINICAL FEATURES

Developmental delay

Child development is a process every child goes through that involves learning and mastering skills such as sitting, walking, talking, skipping and tying shoes. We learn these skills during predictable time periods in our lives and these become known as 'developmental milestones'. Our capabilities mark our developing lives. As parents this is what we look for and are proud of in our children. We also compare our children with other children to gather a general idea of how our children are doing. It is when these milestones are not reached that we begin to question the development of our own child.

There are five main areas of development in children. A child develops the ability to learn and solve problems. A baby learns to explore the environment with hands or eyes or a five-year-old learns how to count and add up. This is cognitive development. A major part of our lives is concerned with others, and children learn to interact socially. Young babies learn to smile in response to their parents and a five-year-old will learn to play games and share toys with other children. This is social and emotional development. Coupled to this social development, children begin to make sounds and vocalisations.

As parents we wait for those first few magical burbles that we take as indications that we are recognised. Later, we hear those other milestones of 'No' and 'Why?' Speech and language development, then, is another feature of the child's progress.

Central to the child developing is the ability to use hands and fingers, to manipulate small objects such as toys and then to hold a spoon. These are the fine motor skills.

As parents, we are continually aware of how our children are developing gross motor skills too. Indeed, we wait eagerly for when they first sit up unaided, the first efforts to crawl, the brave heroics of standing and the first staggering steps. We are also aware when those first events do not materialise. Eventually, we suspect there is a developmental delay, we talk to our family and friends and then contact our physician. While we may have established guidelines, most of us know that our children will have a trajectory of development that is their very own. We also know when something is beginning to go wrong.

Developmental delay in the early years, unless extreme, is not always immediately apparent. Children will develop, even if that development is delayed. That is what we wait for and hope for as parents. Deciding when that development is delayed and a cause for concern is a matter of judgement and not always clear cut.

Hyperactivity

Hyperactivity is a state where the child is abnormally and easily excitable or exuberant, often expressed in strong emotional reactions, impulsive behaviour and sometimes a short span of attention. In other words, a normal terrible two-year-old. So, the feature is not fixed. For hyperactivity in an individual child to be recognised as a disorder, it must be regarded as abnormal by the parents. Again, we usually check this with family and friends and then seek out a professional opinion. Given that young children are by nature active, labelling them as hyperactive is also a matter of judgement, experience and expectation. In Table 3.1 we see the features of a fidgety child, who is constantly 'on the go', disturbs other children and is unruly. All of these features by themselves are not a disorder. All of our children have their moments of restlessness. However, the more of these features that a child shows, collectively, the greater the likelihood that he or she is hyperactive.

BOX 3.1 CHARACTERISTICS OF HYPERACTIVITY

- fidgets or squirms in seat
- repeatedly leaves seat in kindergarten or in other situations where remaining in the seat is expected
- runs about or climbs excessively in situations in which it is inappropriate
- has difficulty playing or engaging in leisure activities quietly
- is often 'on the go'
- often talks excessively
- blurts out answers before questions have been completed
- has difficulty awaiting turns
- often interrupts or intrudes on others
- appears to be restless or unruly.

Short attention span

If a child hasn't learned to listen when someone talks, wait his or her turn, complete a task or return to a task if interrupted, then we begin to think there is a problem with attention. We see in Box 3.2 that many of the features of short attention span would only be recognised once the child is in play school or kindergarten. And, of course, many of these features can be normal characteristics of children less than three or four years old. That is why delay is not immediately apparent. However, if we also see the child as hyperactive – that is, restless, impulsive or always in a hurry – then we are more likely to suspect there is a problem. Some children will have days when all of these features occur. It is when these features become a daily concern that we should consider seeking a professional opinion.

BOX 3.2 CHARACTERISTICS OF SHORT ATTENTION SPAN

- fails to give close attention to details or makes careless mistakes in schoolwork or other activities
- has difficulty sustaining attention in play activities or tasks
- does not seem to listen when directly spoken to
- does not follow through on instructions
- fails to finish schoolwork, chores or duties
- has difficulty organising tasks and activities
- avoids, dislikes or is reluctant to engage in tasks that require sustained mental effort
- loses things necessary for tasks or activities like toys, clothes, pencils or books
- easily distracted by extraneous stimuli
- forgetful in daily activities.

Tactile defensiveness

Some children are sensitive to being touched and avoid touching, or become fearful of situations where they know they will come into contact with either people or materials. As with the previous features, we all see such peculiarities in children without their being a sign of disorder. However, we also know that when these reactions are outside the range of what we expect in a normal child, then something is wrong. Like all things, we only know what is normal by comparing our children with each other, by asking other people who have children of their own and consulting with the child's teachers.

There are many challenging everyday situations for children who experience tactile defensiveness (see Table 3.1), from the simple daily activities of getting washed and dressed to being in the company of family and friends. Children may become anxious or fearful of touch. They may then avoid activities, withdraw or try literally to run away from the situation. For many children with tactile defensiveness, who will only use their fingertips when playing with messy materials, their play opportunities are limited. This limits their ability to learn through experience.

Table 3.1 Characteristics of tactile defensiveness

Sensitive infant	• does not like to be held or cuddled; may arch back, cry and pull away
	• is distressed when nappy is changed
	• avoids touching certain textures of material such as blankets and stuffed animals
	• is distressed by clothes rubbing on skin; toddlers may prefer to be naked or pull nappies and clothes off constantly or may want to wear long-sleeved shirts and long trousers year round to avoid having skin exposed
	• refuses to walk barefoot on grass or sand
	• often walks on tiptoes only
	• is excessively ticklish.

In social situations	• resists friendly or affectionate touch
	• dislikes kisses, will 'wipe off' place where kissed
	• appears fearful of or avoids standing in close proximity to other people or peers
	• avoids group situations for fear of the unexpected touch
	• becomes fearful, anxious or aggressive when touched lightly or unexpectedly.
In play situations	• avoids using hands for play
	• dislikes or avoids 'messy play' in sand, mud and water
	• is distressed by dirty hands and wants to wipe or wash them frequently.
In daily living challenges	• complains about having hair brushed or may demand a particular brush
	• resists having face washed which causes distress
	• resists having hair, toenails or fingernails cut which causes distress
	• resists brushing teeth
	• resists trying new foods; only eats food with certain tastes and textures; mixed textures tend to be avoided as well as hot or cold foods
	• is bothered by rough bed sheets
	• refuses to wear particular clothes with rough textures
	• has adverse reactions or avoidance behaviour in response to wind blowing on the skin or water from the shower
	• overreacts to minor abrasions.

For parents of a baby who is sensitive to touch, the experience of feeding or holding the child becomes extremely challenging.

SPECIFIC FEATURES

The above features of developmental delay, hyperactivity, short attention span and tactile defensiveness are broad in the behaviours that they encompass. Now we turn to a set of characteristics that are more specific and are easier to identify specifically.

Hand flapping

One of the principal themes that we see running through developmental disabilities is that some children are over-sensitive to outside stimuli, as we saw in the section on tactile defensiveness. In addition, some children appear also to be under-sensitive to outside stimuli. What unites these two extremes is children developing a nervous system that has difficulty in managing sensory stimuli, sometimes described as 'sensory integration dysfunction'. Hand flapping is a child's attempt to manage sensory stimuli either by calming him- or herself or integrating sensory stimuli as a connection with the body. This stimulus regulation is often referred to as 'stimming'.

Hand biting

Hand biting can also occur when the child is over-stimulated. Many young children go through a biting phase and that can be troubling for parents. Biting happens for many reasons. Children learn by touching, smelling, hearing and tasting, and biting is another way to explore the world. Biting may be done out of curiosity, but can also be a means of gaining attention and, for the child with a limited means of expression, is a form of expressing frustration. However, biting is also a way of dealing with stress and regulating arousal. Like hand flapping, hand biting is a strategy of arousal regulation and distress management.

Poor eye contact

Eye contact occurs when two peoples look at each other's eyes at the same time. It is a form of intimate non-verbal communication and in Western cultures has a big influence on social behaviour. Eye contact between mother and infant is seen very much as an example of mother–infant bonding. Indeed, eye contact and facial expressions provide important social and emotional information and are also interpreted as signalling attention between those in contact. However, eye contact demands a lot of mental processing either cognitively, for understanding what is going on, or emotionally in terms of arousal. For the infant who is struggling to regulate arousal, eye contact can be a stimulatory challenge that is overwhelming. As with hand biting and hand flapping, avoiding eye contact may be another means of regulating emotional arousal.

Continued repetition of words or phrases

Some children may repeat words or phrases when invited to speak or if asked a question. The repetition of previously heard words or phrases is often termed 'echolalia'. Sometimes words and phrases are repeated immediately or very soon after the original words, or there can be a delay of hours, days or weeks after they were originally heard. Repetition has a communicative function for the child; it may initiate communication or regulate the arousal of communicating itself. Echolalia is a feature of normal language development where the infant repeats what the parents say. In the typically developing child, language is spontaneous and the child repeats what he or she hears with the intention of starting off a communicative dialogue. What we have to remember is that echolalia, the repeating of a word or phrase, has been the stand-by of comedians and television game-show hosts for decades. In religious services, the repetition of phrases is a means of bringing about a change in consciousness, focusing attention and emphasising calm. The same functions can exist for the child: repetition can be calming and stabilising in the face of the challenge that communications brings. Repeated words or phrases are also used in rituals to punctuate the flow of the activity and indicate that something new is to start, such as saying grace before a meal or saying 'thank you' to a speaker who has overrun his allotted time span. The same function may also be ascribed to echolalia. So, the repetition of words has an important function in communication; the exact point at which this turns into the problem of echolalia is a clinical judgement but parents will already be aware that something is not quite right.

Communication is challenging

Communication is an important part of life. We are in constant dialogue with our babies and infants. Yet, for the infant, this can be an enormous challenge. For the infant with a nervous system that is compromised, the challenge can be simply too much. The behaviours mentioned above – hyperactivity, changing attention, hand flapping and biting, avoiding eye contact and repeating words – are ways of trying to regulate the arousal of contact with another person and the environment.

We are alive, so we are constantly aware of what is going on around us and respond to other people and the environment. When we are awake, we are aroused. How that arousal is managed by our nervous system is the basis of whether or not we become pleasantly excited or over-excited. And once we have become excited, then that excitement has to reach its peak and we become calm once more. That is the basis of emotional satisfaction and the way in which we satisfy the desires of everyday life. One of the consequences of Fragile X syndrome is that the way the nervous system works is compromised. It becomes difficult for the child to regulate the necessary arousal he or she needs in everyday life at an acceptable level. Some of the child's behaviours, although at first seeming strange, are attempts at regulating that arousal so that it does not erupt into an overwhelming over-excitement.

Females with full mutations may have a normal IQ, but learning disabilities or emotional problems including social anxiety, selective mutism, shyness, poor eye contact, hyperactivity and impulsive behaviours may be present. Females frequently exhibit only slight cognitive features of the syndrome, such as a difficulty with maths or excessive shyness, without other major effects.

We may see behavioural problems occurring such as depression, obsessive compulsive disorder, impulsiveness, anger outbursts and social anxiety. These too may be reflected in interpersonal relationship difficulties and an inability to adjust to new situations, leading to isolation. In children, we may find temper tantrums, aggressive behaviour, and distractibility that lead us to suspect an underlying problem. The benefit of a genetic understanding demonstrates that these behaviours are not the consequence of a wilful and difficult child, nor a disturbed parental relationship, but based firmly in a genetic and biological substrate. How that child is handled, cared for, educated and loved will change the way in which he or she develops. This is the influence of nurture. But we have to face the fact that many children presenting us with difficulties are doing so through nature. That is the way they are.

PHYSICAL FEATURES

Long face and prominent ears

There are several physical features commonly associated with Fragile X syndrome. Not all children with Fragile X syndrome will exhibit all of these features and these features also appear in some children without Fragile X syndrome.

The primary physical features that people associate with Fragile X syndrome in boys is a long face and prominent ears. These features often become more apparent after the age of ten. The ears may project away from the head and are often wider and longer than usual.

Double-jointedness

There are a number of physical characteristics of persons with Fragile X syndrome that are associated with a connective tissue alteration. Being 'double jointed' means that one has a joint that appears to be unusually flexible. Both boys and girls with Fragile X may be more flexible than is normal and able to hyperextend their elbows, fingers or thumbs; some may be able to bend their knee joints backwards.

Large testicles (macroorchidism)

Macroorchidism (enlarged testicles) is a common feature in adult males who have Fragile X syndrome. Some boys will have macroorchidism before puberty. After puberty, nearly all males will have testicles that are bigger than those of typical normal males.

Other clinical features

Other differences in body structure that we may find are macrocephaly (a large head circumference), a broad forehead and a prominent jaw. Where there is a problem with loose connective tissue we may find flat feet or scoliosis (curvature of the spine). Some children exhibit low muscle tone, mitral valve prolapse (thickening of a heart valve), hernias (where there is a weakening of muscle tissue), strabismus (crossed or 'lazy' eyes) and possibly floppy eustachian tubes leading to recurrent ear infections (otitis media).

Girls with Fragile X syndrome may share some of the physical features that we see in boys, such as long face, long ears, prominent ears and high arched palate, but usually to a lesser degree.

FAMILY HISTORY OF DEVELOPMENTAL DELAY

With Fragile X, as with all genetic disorders, any history of developmental delay in the parents' families it is an important characteristic to take into consideration. We can only discover this history through a careful interview. Sometimes families will be reluctant to talk about such problems, and these problems may have been hidden.

When Rosie came to our centre for help as a teenager because she was being bullied at school, we asked about her family background. Her parents knew already that she had Fragile X syndrome through tests done when she was ten years old. Before that she was considered to have autism. Although behavioural and educational interventions had helped with her autistic features, Rosie was being bullied and becoming withdrawn from her peers and any social contacts. When asked about problems in the family, her mother said there were none, except that she herself had a pre-mutation status for Fragile X and had difficulty conceiving her first child. We now know that this difficulty of conception is also a feature of Primary Ovarian Insufficiency (POI) in female pre-mutated carriers.

During the interview, it also transpired that Rosie's grandfather had been undergoing treatment for dementia for the past five years. No one had made the generational link that the grandfather might also be a pre-mutated carrier, having Fragile X-associated tremor/ataxia syndrome.

As we can imagine, this is a delicate matter. Rosie's case reveals the importance of genetic counselling and uncovering the hidden factors in our families, some of which we may not be aware of, and some of which may have been unwittingly concealed over the years.

We will see in the next chapter how the genetic factors we inherit influence the likelihood of Fragile X syndrome.

Chapter 4

ASSOCIATED FRAGILE X SYNDROMES

Primary Ovarian Insufficiency and Fragile X-associated Tremor/Ataxia Syndrome

We saw in the previous chapter that before the genetic condition of Fragile X reaches a full mutation, there are preliminary stages which we call pre-mutation. The thinking in genetics used to be that for every gene there was a specific function, and a malfunction in that gene would lead to a particular disorder. We now know that the abnormalities work in different ways. If the FMR1 gene is less active than normal then it causes the problem we know as Fragile X syndrome.

As we saw in Chapter 2, when there are more than 200 CGG repeats, then the FMR1 gene is mutated and turned off, or 'silenced', leading to a failure in the production of an important protein for brain development. However, there are situations where the FMR1 gene has between 54 and 200 repeats and this is called the 'pre-mutation stage'. The term pre-mutation is used because it is a condition prior to mutation. It was previously thought that carriers are asymptomatic – that is, without the clinical symptoms of the syndrome, neither physical nor cognitive – because they have a practically normal protein level. Pre-mutated alleles are genetically unstable and can expand in the number of CGG repeats from one generation to another.

This pre-mutation in the FMR1 gene can impair women's ovarian function in the form of Primary Ovarian Insufficiency, which may then cause infertility and early menopause. It can also lead to the syndrome we see as Fragile X-associated tremor/ataxia syndrome (FXTAS) in older adults. So while Fragile X syndrome is due to an absence or deficit of protein, the pre-mutation stages of the same gene can be a result of an abnormal production of messenger RNA (mRNA).

PRIMARY OVARIAN INSUFFICIENCY

Cora visits her gynaecologist. She is 30 years old and has been married for three years. She and her husband want to start a family. However, Cora is having difficulties becoming pregnant and has problems with her periods. Her gynaecologist goes through the normal gynaecological tests and Cora is diagnosed as having an ovarian insufficiency. Cora is distressed at this news. Her gynaecologist suggests in-vitro fertilisation. Her ovaries are stimulated hormonally to release eggs and finally she becomes successfully pregnant through in-vitro fertilisation using the sperm of her husband. Twins are born: a boy and a girl. Time passes and it becomes apparent that the little boy is not developing at the same rate as his sister.

The concerned parents consult different paediatricians, one of whom suggests that they perform a genetic test on the boy. He is by now two years old. The diagnosis is Fragile X syndrome and the parents are referred to a genetic counsellor. Cora is shocked when she realises that she was a pre-mutated carrier of Fragile X and the full syndrome in her little boy could have been avoided. Reproductive difficulties like hers are a frequent feature of female pre-mutated carriers. If her gynaecologist had been aware of this, he could have suggested using alternative treatment (see pp.58–60 for the options available).

Originally, the term Premature Ovarian Failure (POF) was used to describe the condition now known as Primary Ovarian Insufficiency (POI), but the term 'failure' has negative connotations and implies that women with this diagnosis will not become pregnant, when in fact 5–10 per cent of these women do get pregnant. We now use POI as a more accurate medical term for this condition, in which the ovaries stop functioning normally in a woman younger than age 40.

The common symptoms of POI include absent or irregular periods and infertility but it is not menopause, though the symptoms, such as menstrual irregularity, hot flashes and vaginal dryness, may be similar. 'Menopause' is defined as a permanent or total cessation of the monthly period or menstruation, which is not always the case with POI. There may also be a return of menstrual periods so that some of these women may become pregnant because their ovaries function intermittently to release viable eggs.

In normal ovarian function, women will experience regular menstrual cycles. Part of this cycle will not only be the release of eggs but also of the hormones oestrogen and progesterone. Abnormalities in the FRM1 gene, the pre-mutation, can be associated with problems in this cyclical ovarian function and hormonal alteration. Young women who notice a change from their normal menstrual cycle should visit their gynaecologist who will recommend an hormone test.

It is necessary to keep in mind that women with the pre-mutation cannot assume that they have reduced fertility or that they are infertile. Pregnancy can occur, even though fertility may be reduced. Studies show that some women with the FMR1 pre-mutation experience early menopause. Normal menopause, the permanent cessation of menstrual periods, occurs on average when a woman is between 45 and 55 years old. Early menopause is defined as occurring before the age of 40.

On the cognitive behavioural and emotional level there may be a predisposition to depression in women with pre-mutation, independent of their life situation. This means not only do women suffer the emotional burden of having a child with a disability, but they may also have a predisposition to depression. Women carrying the pre-mutation without children, or prior to having them, can also be susceptible to depression. Social anxiety and timidity may also be problems for a number of women with pre-mutation, although having normal cognitive abilities helps them to overcome their problems and cope. Some women with pre-mutation are also defined as impulsive and particularly active. These traits can be converted into positive features for mothers, resulting in a strong fighting spirit where they work consistently for the future and well-being of their children.

Women who have POI have a 1 in 50 chance of being a carrier of the FMR1 gene pre-mutation. If there is also a family history of female relatives with POI then the risk rises to a 1 in 15 chance of carrying this pre-mutation. The percentage of women presenting with POI is bigger when there is an increased number of CGG repeats. This risk begins to decrease after 100 CGG repeats in the allele. We know that for carriers of the FMR1 pre-mutation there is a significant risk of having a child with Fragile X syndrome, so testing for the FMR1 pre-mutation is recommended in women with POI.

Women with full mutation may never present POI and have absolutely normal ovarian functions. It is extremely useful for women with pre-mutation to know if they will have POI or not, in order to plan their reproductive lives, to receive genetic counselling and to avoid possible unwanted pregnancies.

FRAGILE X-ASSOCIATED TREMOR/ATAXIA SYNDROME

Oscar visits his doctor. He is 64 years old and is concerned about a tremor in his hand when he reaches out for anything. He has fallen recently and, as he says, he is not so steady on his feet as he was. Eventually, after a long referral process, he is diagnosed as being in the early onset stages of Parkinson's disease. A few months later, his first grandson Albert is born and his daughter Mary is overjoyed at the birth following a complicated history of trying to become pregnant. One year later, Mary is concerned about Albert. He does not appear to be doing the things a baby should be doing at one year of age even though his paediatrician says that some babies are slower to develop than others. Months later, her concerns are strengthened and the paediatrician decides to check Albert regarding Fragile X. The test result is positive; Albert has a full mutation in the FMR1 gene. A referral to a genetic counsellor takes place and the family members are also tested for Fragile X. Oscar, the grandfather, is discovered to have a pre-mutation in the FMR1 gene. The ramification of this discovery for Oscar is that his neurologist can now change his diagnosis from early onset Parkinson's disease to that of

FXTAS. Mary is also found to be a pre-mutation carrier and this could have been the reason for her reproductive difficulties.

If Oscar had been tested earlier, Mary could have known her genetic status and attended a genetic counsellor to discuss her reproductive choices.

FXTAS is a relatively new syndrome and consists of a multisystemic neurological disorder with tremor and ataxia as its main signs. This occurs in patients carrying the pre-mutation but not in patients with full mutation. Until a few years ago, patients with pre-mutation were considered free from clinical pathology but FXTAS is now considered to be a new entity related to pre-mutation.

The ataxia in FXTAS is characterised by a difficulty in walking, which may be associated with miscalculating distances, and difficulties in articulating words. The majority of patients with FXTAS present difficulties in walking and in coordinating steps, which provoke frequent falls. They may therefore need some type of walking aid.

About 90 per cent of those affected by FXTAS also present intentional tremor. It usually starts in the dominant hand and, with time, affects both hands. An 'intentional tremor' is a tremor that occurs when reaching for an object, as opposed to a tremor that appears when a person is at rest. In general it progresses over the years and finally affects daily activities.

Other pathological characteristics associated with ataxia and tremor

We also find the following symptoms of Parkinsonism in FXTAS: bradykinesia (slowed down movements), rigidity (mainly in the upper arm) and instability of balance. The instability while walking may result in patients walking with their feet farther apart, which itself influences their gait. Fourteen per cent of FXTAS patients have been described as having a family history of Parkinson's disease, which is why it may be confused with Parkinson's disease. They may also have dystonia (alterations of muscle tone).

Diagnosis of FXTAS

The foremost requirement for the diagnosis of FXTAS is a genetic test. A definitive diagnosis is made when apart from the state of pre-mutation in FMR1 the patient presents a principal radiological sign linked to ataxia and/or intentional tremor. The diagnosis is considered probable when in addition to the principal radiological criterion there is another minor clinical sign (see Table 4.1).

Meanwhile, the first cases of FXTAS in women have been described. To date, none of them has been associated with dementia, which has been described in males with FXTAS. This may be due to the presence of two X chromosomes in females or to the effects of female hormones.

Table 4.1 Clinical signs of FXTAS

1a Principal clinical signs:	i) intentional tremor in men aged 50 years or over
	ii) ataxia.
1b Minor clinical signs:	i) Parkinsonism
	ii) moderate to grave deficit in short-term memory
	iii) deficit in executive function.
2a Principal radiological signs:	i) lesions in the white substance of the penduculum cerebellum.
2b Less frequent radiological signs:	i) lesions of the white brain substance
	ii) moderate to grave brain atrophy.

Source: Hagerman, R., Hall, D., Coffey, S., Leehey, M. *et al.* (2008) 'Treatment of fragile X-associated tremor ataxia syndrome (FXTAS) and related neurological problems.' *Clinical Interventions in Aging 3*, 2, 251–62.

Prevalence

The prevalence of FXTAS in males over 50 years is approximately 1 in 3000 in the general population. This figure suggests that this syndrome is one of the most frequent genetic causes of tremor and ataxia in adults. We estimate that approximately 1 in 100 to 260 females and 1 in 260 to 800 males carry a pre-mutation of the Fragile X gene. The chances of developing the core symptoms of FXTAS in male pre-mutation carriers increases incrementally with age. As we saw, the estimate for males over 50 years of age is approximately 17 per cent and this rises to 75 per cent in men over 80 years.

FXTAS is associated with an increase in messenger ribonucleic acid (mRNA) in brain cells that appears to have a toxic effect.

To find out if a family member has the syndrome, it is necessary to make a diagnosis based on three factors:

- first, a neurological examination to confirm the symptomatic observations

- second, magnetic resonance imaging (MRI) which will discover changes that are known to be related to Fragile X-associated tremor/ataxia syndrome, including white matter changes or other alterations of the brain

- third, a genetic test that ascertains that the person is a positive carrier of the FMR1 pre-mutation.

It is important that a genetic assessment is made of elderly persons with ataxia and intentional tremor to discover if there is an expansion of the FMR1 gene, particularly if there are additional clinical features such as Parkinsonism or loss of cognitive function.

Chapter 5

DIAGNOSING FRAGILE X SYNDROME AND ITS IMPLICATIONS

The clinical manifestations of Fragile X syndrome are variable, depending on age and gender, so a clinical diagnosis from appearances and behaviour is always difficult. As we saw in previous chapters, there are recognisable physical and behavioural features associated with Fragile X syndrome, but these are not always present. The result is that Fragile X syndrome may not be diagnosed simply from clinical signs. This is even more the case in females with Fragile X syndrome as the presentation of the condition can be much more subtle.

A clinical test can be useful as a preliminary screening (see Table 5.1) but clinical diagnosis has to be confirmed by a genetic test. The diagnosis of Fragile X syndrome requires the detection of an alteration in the FMR1 gene at Xq27.3.

TESTING FOR FRAGILE X

Originally Fragile X syndrome was diagnosed by a chromosome test developed by Herbert Lubs 1969.[1] This chromosome or cytogenetic test has now been replaced by more accurate molecular tests. With the discovery of the FMR1 gene in 1991, molecular tests were introduced for detecting

---

1   Lubs, H.A. (1969) 'A marker X-chromosome.' *American Journal of Human Genetics 21*, 231–244.

Table 5.1 Fragile X syndrome clinical checklist

		Scores		
		0	**1**	**2**
Intellectual disability	IQ>85	70–85	<70	
Family history of developmental delay	no	history of depression in mother's family	history of developmental delay in mother's family	
Hyperactivity and short attention span	no	only hyperactivity	yes, both	
Elongated face	no	questionable	yes	
Autistic features: hand flapping, hand biting, poor eye contact, continued repetitions of words or phrases, responds negatively to touch (tactile defensiveness)	no	one of the features	several of the features	
Large or prominent ears	no	questionable	yes	
Total scores *		0	1	2

* If the score is more than 5 then a confirmatory molecular test is suggested.

Source: Fernández, I., Tellería, J.J., Blanco, A., Alonso, M.J. *et al.* (2001) 'Effectiveness of a clinical test in the preselection of children with suspected fragile X syndrome.' *Anales de Pediatría* 54, 4, 227–31.

Fragile X. This DNA testing is considered to be the most accurate way of ascertaining genetic status.

The methods for molecular Fragile X diagnosis are PCR (polymerase chain reaction) and Southern Blot analysis. Combining both methodologies, testing is 99 per cent sensitive in detecting affected and carrier individuals. Only on rare occasions is an individual who has Fragile X syndrome missed because a mutation other than CGG expansion has occurred.

A blood sample is needed to make a molecular test. DNA is isolated from white blood cells in the laboratory to perform the PCR test or Southern Blot analysis.

The Fragile X DNA test has revolutionised diagnosis with strong implications for genetic counselling. As a test, it is reliable for people of any age. It can also be performed before and during pregnancy. Foetal testing performed on amniotic fluid cells or placental tissue is also available when a parent is a known carrier.

A positive FMR1 test result is considered to be 100 per cent certain.

What is tested?

When a molecular test is carried out for the Fragile X mutation it measures the length of the FMR1 gene region containing the CGG repeat stretch and then calculates the CGG repeat number by PCR analysis and/or analysis of the gene's methylation status by Southern Blot analysis (that is, whether the gene is turned 'off' or 'on'). Knowing the number of CGG repeats is useful for genetic counselling in pre-mutation carriers.

Sometimes there are different-sized CGG repeat expansions in different populations of blood cells. This is known as 'size mosaicism'. We may also find methylation mosaicism in full-mutated carriers where some cells do indeed make FMRP (the protein associated with Fragile X syndrome). This means we have to be careful in interpreting results in terms of understanding what the consequences will be for the development of the child. While we may know the exact status of the genetic change, we cannot say how this will influence the child's development. We all have our own genetic constitution but this is influenced by the environment in which we develop. In technical terms this is called the phenotype. In the presence of mosaicism, it is even harder to predict what influence this will have upon the child's development and problems may be less severe.

When to test

If you are considering a test for Fragile X syndrome, then it is important to consider the circumstances. No one undertakes such a test lightly as the consequences are potentially life changing for the child, for the parents, for the wider family and for coming generations. That is what genetics is about: our very identity and what is passed on to the next generation. We can only emphasise here that it is important to contact a genetic counsellor as soon as possible in this process.

If you are concerned about your child, then you have probably seen some of the behavioural or physical characteristics we mentioned earlier. You need to visit your doctor to discuss this and consider a DNA test (see Box 5.1).

It may be that there is a family history of developmental disability of some kind and there are concerns that there is a risk for any children in the future. Specific indications for testing are the presence of any male or female with developmental delay or learning disabilities of unknown cause, the presence of autism or autistic-like characteristics, a relative who has Fragile X syndrome or intellectual disability of unknown cause and any previous positive or equivocal result from the Fragile X cytogenetic test.

BOX 5.1 WHEN TO CONDUCT A GENETIC TEST

- if the child shows evidence of developmental delay or intellectual disability, or exhibits autistic features
- if any family member has developmental delay, intellectual disability or learning problems with an unknown cause
- if any family member has autistic features
- if female relatives have a history of ovarian insufficiency or premature menopause
- if men and women over the age of 50 have intentional tremor, ataxia or symptoms of Parkinsonism.

The carriers of Fragile X syndrome may be unaware that they are carriers as they are usually asymptomatic and there may not be a family history of Fragile X syndrome, or, if there is a family member with Fragile X syndrome, he or she may not have been previously diagnosed. As the carrier rate in females is quite high, at approximately 1 in 300, it is recommended that Fragile X carrier testing be offered to all women of reproductive age who have a relative with developmental delay of unknown cause. Molecular tests for pre-mutation should be performed in elderly people with ataxia and intentional tremor because, as we have seen, the prevalence rises sharply after the age of 50 years.

A physician, or other appropriate health care professional, is the person who calls for the test and receives the results of the test from the laboratory. If you want a test for yourself or someone in your family then you should ask your family physician to refer you to a clinical geneticist or genetic counsellor. If you are concerned about the signs we mentioned earlier, then you will have already contacted your child's paediatrician who can arrange a test.

Whenever the diagnosis of Fragile X syndrome is confirmed in a boy, then the mother and one of the maternal grandparents are carriers. When it is confirmed in a girl, then either mother or father could be the carrier. The brothers or sisters of the carrier parent and the brothers or sisters of the affected patient have a 50 per cent risk of being carriers. The ideal way to find this out is to consult a genetic service, and then the expert will discuss with you, on the basis of the family tree, which family members are at risk of being carriers, and if and when they should be tested.

It is understandable that when families are confronted with such a diagnosis and receive a confirmation of the condition then they may feel emotionally overwhelmed by the complexity of the disorder and the implications this has for the family. This is where genetic counsellors are important in advising about the genetics of the condition and implications for other family members. Counsellors offer ongoing support prior to and during testing, throughout the process of making decisions based on the results of testing, and into the future.

The female carriers of the pre-mutation must be informed of the risk of reduced fertility, since this has implications for the age at which they might try to conceive children, and impacts on the decision of whether to have prenatal or pre-implantational diagnosis.

REPRODUCTIVE OPTIONS OFFERED TO KNOWN CARRIERS

There are several reproductive options for pre-mutation or full mutation carriers who wish to have children and we would recommend immediate support by a geneticist in all cases.

Donation of gametes: ovules or sperm

This is an increasingly accepted technique, above all in the case of donation of ovules, and has a very high success rate. The mother experiences her pregnancy in exactly the same way as any other mother, it is strictly confidential, and we would only recommend that the donor is checked explicitly in regard of Fragile X syndrome, since 1 among 300 females of the general population is a carrier. Sperm donors should also be screened in order to avoid a male with pre-mutation having daughters who carry the pre-mutation.

Pre-implantational and pre-conceptional diagnostics

Pre-implantational genetic diagnosis (PGD) is a diagnostic technique based on the genetic analysis of an embryo obtained by in-vitro fertilisation and the subsequent transfer of the genetically healthy and viable embryos.

Pre-conceptional diagnosis (PCD) is based on the genetic study of the ovule prior to fertilisation and the subsequent in-vitro fertilisation of healthy ovules.

Both techniques basically have the same advantages and drawbacks.

Diagnostics prior to pregnancy avoid stress, emotional trauma and the moral dilemma of a voluntary interruption of the pregnancy, since only healthy embryos are implanted (no carriers, no affected children); they lead to a reduction in the incidence of the syndrome. One disadvantage is that it is necessary to have in-vitro fertilisation performed, in which at best only 30 per cent of transfers are successful. While this method sounds simple when written, it is complicated in reality. For all these reasons, only very few centres offer these procedures to date. However, with the advances in this field, and a great demand from the families concerned, there may be significant advances in the near future.

Ovarian insufficiency, which affects over 20 per cent of females with pre-mutation, reduces the efficiency of the in-vitro fertilisation, quite apart from the numerous technical problems the procedure involves. In any case a prenatal diagnosis must be recommended in order to confirm the results.

Prenatal diagnostics

Prenatal diagnostics of Fragile X syndrome is an invasive method by amniocentesis. Under amniocentesis, a small amount of amniotic fluid, which contains foetal tissues, is extracted from the amniotic sac surrounding a developing foetus, and the foetal DNA examined for genetic abnormalities. Placental tissue sampling entails taking a sample of the chorionic villus and testing it. Placental tissue sampling can be carried out 10–12 weeks after the last period, which is earlier than amniocentesis (which is carried out at 16–20 weeks). The problem with chorionic villus sampling is that chemical changes (methylation status) in the placental tissue are incomplete at 10–12 weeks and there can be a problem in interpreting the analysis results and their implications for the eventual clinical status.

Prenatal diagnostics are offered to women carrying the premutation or full mutation. This information is intended to facilitate the decision-making process for potential parents and, ultimately, to prepare them for being confronted with a positive result (that there is a genetic mutation).

✳ The diagnosis of Fragile X syndrome implies better treatment for the patient, which contributes to improved prognostics. For the family, it provides access to appropriate information, an efficient planning of their reproductive future, and also access to support groups or organisations.

Chapter 6

INTERVENTIONS FOR FRAGILE X SYNDROME

As we have seen in the previous chapters, Fragile X syndrome is the most common cause of inherited neurodevelopmental disability.

While our knowledge of genetics has increased substantially in the last ten years, and we know more about the Fragile X gene mutation and its consequence – an absence of a protein that itself regulates other proteins in the brain – the results of this protein change are complex. At this time there is no cure. But, help is at hand. The good news is that with our increased knowledge of genetics there has been a dramatic increase in therapeutic developments, extending the existing knowledge base in clinical practice. The key to any treatment is multidisciplinarity; counsellors, psychologists, educationalists, occupational therapists and medical practitioners all have something valuable to offer. There is an emerging call for these practitioners to work together with research scientists to bring new treatments to families.

Treatment strategies are improving and there are extensive support networks. There are a variety of ways to help minimise the symptoms of the condition; drugs therapies that may improve attention impairment and hyperactivity are available. We cannot repeat often enough, the most important thing we can do is to establish an early multidisciplinary intervention with therapies, including speech, physical, psychological and music therapies, that will all provide real benefit to people with the syndrome. As a parent or caregiver of someone with Fragile X syndrome, the challenge will be to become aware of and then coordinate these possibilities. This is no mean feat. Coordinating them is often a challenge but you will not need them all at one time. Perhaps most importantly, there are networks of self-help associations in most countries with sound expertise that you can call upon from parents who have had similar experiences to yours.

. It is important to remember that Fragile X is not like a childhood infectious disease that can be treated simply with medication like an antibiotic. In the treatment of Fragile X, as in autism spectrum disorders, we can offer medications that attempt to alleviate some of the symptoms, and modify behaviour, but we cannot offer one medication that solves the problem by removing the cause. The problem is the disruption of the necessary proteins for facilitating connections between nerve cells in the brain. While investigators and pharmaceutical firms are going ahead with exciting research into medications that mediate these connections, none of these products are yet available for specific treatments.

Fragile X is a syndrome. This means that, by its very nature, it is an aggregate of symptoms that happen together. The consequences of the genetic changes will be shown differently in each child.

Currently treatments are symptom-oriented (see Box 6.1). An improvement of symptoms means an improved quality of life for the affected child and for the family. Medications are used to treat many of the symptoms associated with Fragile X, but because they lack specificity, it is important to accompany them with behavioural and educational interventions. As this is a lifelong problem, any treatment strategies will vary according to the way in which the child develops.

Although Fragile X is described as a developmental disability, it is important to remember that all children develop at different rates. Each child is unique in the way that the Fragile X syndrome expresses itself, and the consequences of the genetic disorder will be different for each child and confounded by what is a complex clinical picture. We know the syndrome is a complex of symptoms that develop over time and that medication, while altering one aspect, may disturb another aspect. Once we enter the realm of altering brain chemistry at an early age, we have to be very aware of the consequences of those alterations.

Studies are taking place throughout the world looking at specific treatments. It has been suggested that mGluR5 antagonists could be an effective treatment for Fragile X syndrome and these have been tested extensively in animal models. Some of these drugs are under development as an orphan drug (a pharmaceutical agent that has been developed specifically to treat a rare medical condition) for the treatment of Fragile X syndrome, with initial human Fragile X syndrome trials recently taking place, so we expect positive results in the near future. How near that future is in terms of registered products is impossible to say.

BOX 6.1 SOURCES OF SPECIALIST PROFESSIONAL HELP

- Family doctor or paediatrician for a general overview and for dealing with problems such as gastrooesophageal reflux, sinusitis and otitis media.

- Genetic counsellor, particularly for family planning decisions.

- Special education professional to assess cognitive functioning, attention deficit hyperactivity and aggressiveness, and to initiate sensory integration therapy for behaviour problems.

- Psychologist or behavioural specialist is important in suggesting methods for coping with negative behaviour. Some patients benefit from learning social skills and individual counselling. This may also include behavioural intervention/modification for reducing social anxiety.

- Neurologist, particularly if there is a problem with seizures and for older pre-mutated carriers.

- Cardiologist for mitral valve prolapse and heart problems in general.

- Ophthalmologist for problems with crossed or 'lazy eyes'.

- Orthopaedic surgeon if there is a problem with flat feet or scoliosis.

- Speech and language therapist with a specialist knowledge of Fragile X problems for working with speech and language.

- Music therapist for promoting non-verbal communication.

- Occupational and physical therapist with specialist knowledge of working with sensory integration methods and for improving gross and fine motor skills.

Not every medication will help every patient with symptoms related to Fragile X in the same way. It is between you and your doctor to decide what medicines your child needs and, if prescribed, how the dosage will be adjusted. A drug may be effective for a certain period but this does not mean that it will continue to be so for the child's lifetime. Your doctor may have to adjust the dose more precisely for the child and this means periodical checks. While there are positive benefits from some medication, it is the side effects that are the main problem, particularly when medication is used over the long term.

BEHAVIOURAL FEATURES

The behavioural phenotype of Fragile X syndrome involves anxiety, attention deficits, hyperactivity, impulsivity, hyperarousal to sensory stimuli, poor eye contact, excessive shyness, hand flapping, hand biting, aggression, tactile defensiveness and cognitive development.

Anxiety

Anxiety is based on two important factors. First is the ability of the child to regulate his or her own emotions and an ability to pick up clues from the behaviour of others for how to regulate behaviour. Normally, the child does this naturally from birth relying on the tone of the mother's voice, how she moves and particularly from her facial expressions. Second, the mother watches the child's face for his or her expressions, sees how he or she moves in coordination with her and listens to the sounds he or she makes. Both these factors are coordinated in mother–child interaction but are dependent upon the child's sensory networks being intact and functioning. Many of the problems that we see both in Fragile X syndrome and in autism spectrum disorders are based on the difficulties that the child faces in coordinating his or her behaviour with, first, the mother, and then other people. This is nothing to do with the behaviour of the mother, but is purely a result of how the child regulates his or her own emotions and enters the ecology of the communicative world, which is dependent on a vast complex of neurological signalling processes. In addition, other people have difficulty in coordinating their responses with the child appropriately. Small wonder that this results in social anxiety that we locate in the child rather than in the situation itself.

Some effective drugs, such as selective serotonin reuptake inhibitors (SSRIs) and fluoxetine, have been used for the treatment of anxiety. The important thing is to consult with your doctor and make a careful treatment plan that is suited to your child. There is no one medical intervention that will fit all children. Most practitioners will discuss with you the appropriate dosage for relieving your child's symptoms and a suitable behavioural intervention strategy.

Attention deficits and hyperactivity

Attention deficits and hyperactivity are often seen in younger patients with Fragile X syndrome and are a major source of requests for medication. Paradoxically, stimulants like methylphenidate (with the commercial names of Ritalin®, Concerta® and Rubifen®) have been one of the first choice treatments. We say paradoxically, because it seems counter-intuitive to prescribe a stimulant to a child already being described as hyperactive. The reason this treatment can be effective is that the child is stimulated enough to focus on the task in hand.

Stimulants are commonly used in boys with Fragile X syndrome even before a diagnosis is made. In general, children with Fragile X syndrome are sensitive to stimulants, and their mood often becomes brittle, with an increase in outbursts at higher doses. The side effects of stimulant medication include appetite suppression with possible weight loss, which, when excessive, can decrease height growth. The cardiovascular system is also stimulated, including heart rate and blood pressure. Children on stimulant medication should be seen by their physicians to check their arterial tension and heart rate.

Treatment of attention deficit and hyperactivity symptoms in younger children with non-stimulant medications may be helpful. Adrenergic receptor antagonists including clonidine and guanfacine and sometimes L-acetyl-carnitine seem to be a reasonable alternative. Again, it is only your doctor who can advise you on medication. Remember, you too are an expert on your child and know what is benefiting him or her. All medications have side-effects, and it is important to discuss them with your doctor. It is also important to collaborate actively with your doctor to discuss your observations, express your doubts and offer suggestions. There are many educational and psychological behavioural interventions for coping with hyperactivity and attention deficit, so it is important to talk with teachers and psychologists to find a treatment plan tailored to fit the needs of your child.

Aggression and mood instability

Antipsychotic drugs generally are helpful in clinical settings to target irritability, aggression, mood instability and perseverative behaviours in both male and female individuals with Fragile X syndrome. Risperidone is the most frequently used antipsychotic drug.

Taking the decision to use these drugs with your child needs considerable forethought. While symptoms can be managed in the short term, the decision to use such medication that may continue over a long term is a major decision when we think about the consequences for the developing brain of the child.

Arousal

What we believe to be important in this debate is a wider consideration of how a child manages arousal. Arousal is a physiological and psychological state of being awake or reactive to stimuli. There are many different neural systems involved in being aroused and these include the brain's neurotransmitters. When these systems are in action, the receiving neural areas become sensitive and responsive to incoming signals. It is these areas that are functionally disturbed in Fragile X syndrome. As a result, arousal becomes unregulated.

Arousal is important in regulating consciousness, attention and information processing and, particularly where Fragile X children are concerned, in regulating emotions. When children are aroused in social situations, or when they are being touched, or when they need to communicate, their behaviour appears to be abnormal. Many of the symptoms of Fragile X syndrome can be seen as a difficulty in regulating arousal. Once we see these symptoms as behavioural attempts by children to manage their own situational arousal, then we can begin to find suitable interventions. Rather than see naughty, difficult or wilful children, we can simply see children coming to terms with themselves in response to the situation that they are in. We can then take steps to influence the environment in those cycles of regulation. One means is medication that changes the internal environment of the child. Another way is to change the external environment for the child.

Some authors suggest that children with attention deficit hyperactivity disorder (ADHD) seek self-stimulation or excessive activity in order to transcend their state of abnormally low arousal. If children cannot regulate themselves, then they can only be regulated by environmental stimuli. This explains compulsive hyperactive behaviour as a chronic state of stimulus-hunger, in which they need more external stimulation to feel normal. Without enough stimulation coming from the environment, children will create it for themselves by walking around, fidgeting, talking or making noises. This theory has been used to explain why stimulant medications have high success rates and can induce a calming effect. People with autism explain their own stereotypical behaviour, such as 'stimming', as a means of regulating their own reactions to external stimuli.

What unites both of these perspectives is that arousal has to be regulated within parameters that are comfortable within the child and not cause excess anxiety which is then exhibited in unacceptable behaviours.

Cognitive development

Many persons with Fragile X syndrome have some cognitive weaknesses that appear as problems in thinking, problem solving, concept understanding, information processing and overall intelligence. However, children still have patterns of strengths and weaknesses in their development and may do very well with certain types of learning.

Up to 80 per cent of males with Fragile X syndrome are considered to be cognitively delayed. With an increased awareness of Fragile X, the diagnosis of Fragile X syndrome has improved and 10–15 per cent of the boys tested have IQs in the borderline or mild mental retardation range.

Many boys, and some girls, are described as having a non-progressive disorder that becomes evident during childhood, with disabilities in adapting to the environment and a score on an IQ test below 70. Scores in the mental retardation range may be in the mild range (55–69 IQ), moderate (40–54), severe (25–39) or profound (less than 25). Children with Fragile X syndrome move forward in their development but at a slower pace, and with a lower end result, than normally developing children do. Cognition is also affected by ADHD, seizure disorders, anxiety, speech and language disorders, sensory motor problems and other issues that may impact both test taking and learning. Many children with Fragile X achieve more than would be expected based upon their IQ scores.

Behaviour characteristics in children

Children with Fragile X syndrome are described as sweet and loving with a strong desire for social interactions and often having a good sense of humour. Musical play resources are ideal for such children and interaction is at the heart of music therapy.

Children with Fragile X also often have a variety of behavioural challenges. Behavioural challenges are one of the main areas listed on checklists for the identification of persons with Fragile X syndrome.

A high number of boys with Fragile X are described as distractible and impulsive, with symptoms of ADHD or attention deficit disorder (ADD). They may have short attention spans and difficulty staying on task. Girls tend to show less hyperactivity.

Many boys have unusual, stereotypic behaviours, such as hand flapping and chewing on skin, clothing or objects, which may be connected to sensory processing problems and anxiety. Sensory processing problems may manifest themselves as tactile defensiveness, including oral motor defensiveness, sensitivity to sound or light and poor eye contact.

Anxiety in both boys and girls manifests itself in various ways. Some persons with Fragile X become very worried about changes in routine or upcoming stressful events, a condition known as 'hypervigilance'. Some children become rigid and tense. Sometimes, children simply tighten up their hands, throw temper tantrums or have a feeling of being overwhelmed in certain situations.

Many of the behaviour problems of both boys and girls with Fragile X syndrome also overlap with pragmatic conversational difficulties of language. The poor eye contact and difficulty sustaining a conversation cause many social weaknesses. Perseverative speech and self-talk may be symptoms of anxiety. It is the prosodic speech elements of language and particularly dialogue that music therapy addresses. One of the difficulties of talking about language and language acquisition is that it sounds as if language is a thing in itself to be had. The process of doing language is complex but predominantly a social activity of communication.

Some behaviours that overlap with the diagnosis of autism are often reported. The majority of children with Fragile X syndrome do not have all the characteristics of autism, but about 15–33 per cent are diagnosed as autistic. More often, children have 'autistic-like' features, such as poor eye contact, hand flapping and poor social skills.

BEHAVIOURAL INTERVENTIONS

Behavioural interventions for the treatment and management of children with intellectual disabilities have been successful in improving social skills, communication and intellectual and adaptive functioning. As in the medication studies mentioned previously, the behavioural studies that have taken place have been small scale. Problems related to sleeping difficulties and toilet training have responded well to behavioural interventions.

It is perhaps unlikely that a single medication will improve intellectual and adaptive functioning in Fragile X syndrome. Even if a medication could eradicate the deleterious effects of reduced FMRP in the brain, educational learning programmes will still be needed to develop basic skill sets that have been missed. We recommend early interventions to promote communication, enhance self-regulation and promote new skills. Because these interventions are individualised and labour intensive they may be costly, but they are invaluable. There is, however, a need for more professionals to be trained to be aware of and skilled in meeting the needs of children with developmental disability.

Children do develop despite their challenges. Research on child development among all types of children points to the importance of the early years for encouraging that development. For children with Fragile X syndrome, these early years are of vital importance for stimulating maximum learning, enhancing communication and regulating anxiety.

MUSIC AS AN INTERVENTION

We know music works in social and educational integration, emotional regulation, sensory coordination and in promoting communication through speech and language. Because of the challenge to the developing neural networks of the child's brain, it is important to stimulate sensory integration in a structured way. We do this naturally with our children when we sing and play with them by offering them a communication that is structured in time, restricted in its content and repetitious; that is, the classic children's play song, lullaby or nursery rhyme. From birth, the child becomes accustomed to the mother's voice and the musical elements of speech before he or she can understand the words beings spoken. It is this musical structure that is primary in facilitating communication. One of the bases of musical structure is timing. In the communications between mother and child the communication is dependent upon a mutual timing. In this way, we support our babies to communicate with us, just as they support us to communicate with them. Indeed, communication is a property of the relationship itself. We communicate efficiently when we coordinate the timing of the sounds we make, our facial expressions and the ways in which we react to what the other person says and does. We know that if there is the slightest delay neurologically in the perception of a sound that is related to an action, then children become disorientated both in time and space.

For the child, timing is important for sensory coordination. The child learns that his or her movements, the sounds that he or she makes, his or her facial expressions and the posture of his or her body are expressive.

Help is best provided in an appropriate social setting that does not focus on specific pathologies but emphasises competencies. The needs of these children in terms of social reciprocity or responsiveness, improved language and communication skills, and an enhanced repertoire of activities and interests can be met in a cultural setting. Children with Fragile X syndrome develop but at a slower pace and with a lower end result than do normally developing children. Disabilities in adapting to the environment refer to delays in life skills and not just academic skills.

Music, through singing and play songs, promotes communication, particularly verbal skills through social interaction. Through singing and active music making, musical resources also promote attention and encourage interpersonal reactions that involve personalised, sequenced, structured activities. Music activities, by their very nature, concentrate on sensory integration, regulate arousal levels and encourage fine motor skills.

Daily living skills

Daily living skills are all of the areas of development that are integral to our everyday routines. Eating, sleeping, dressing, washing and bathing, taking care of hygiene and toileting are all daily living skills that may provide challenges for children and adults with Fragile X syndrome and their families.

On the basis of symptoms determined by child psychiatrists, paediatricians, psychologists and neurologists, it is possible to create individually based therapeutic programmes that include a range of therapeutic interventions. We suggest that these include musical play and music therapy. Such programmes require an appropriate integrated treatment setting.

We know that children with Fragile X syndrome have unique speech and language disorders, especially regarding pragmatics. Speech and language are also affected by physical, oral-motor, attention and behavioural characteristics. An integrated approach including music concentrates on establishing dialogue between participants. To do this we encourage mothers and babies to vocalise together, to sing in a structured form (as songs) and to interact in a time-structured format (play songs). Play songs, lullabies and rhyming games are evident in almost every culture, so the intervention can also be adapted to ethnic origin. Furthermore, music therapy specifically uses extant vocalisation as the basis for improvised dialogue with young children. Essentially we concentrate on potential and capabilities and build upon these.

For children who have difficulty in pragmatic speech, with anxiety and shyness affecting their social interactions, music making, through singing and play songs, promotes communication, and particularly verbal skills through social interaction.

Behaviour disorders

Many of the behavioural problems of Fragile X patients are really the consequence of the child not being able to regulate his or her emotions or activity. Like all things, this personal control does not occur in isolation and impinges on the caregivers. Indeed, parents of babies and small infants with Fragile X find that they have difficulty in regulating their child. As we saw, no one is to blame; what has happened is that there has been a genetic change and this has influenced the way in which the brain and nervous system function in response to being stimulated. Communication between parents and the child is absolutely central to their relationship; if that breaks down early on then development is challenged and this also has ramifications for learning both at home and at school.

Children with Fragile X often have a variety of behavioural challenges and these include difficulties with attention, anxiety and interpersonal relations. Parents and educators need to devise behavioural plans to help children with Fragile X to cope with the everyday demands of home, school and community. Poor eye contact, hand flapping and lack of awareness of social cues may cause difficulties in peer interactions, making inclusive educational placements more of a challenge. ADHD may also impede academic progress.

By using individually composed songs for children related to the steps of social routines we can help children to cope with those routines such as entering the classroom, greeting the teacher and/or peers and engaging in play.

For young children with autism enrolled in community-based inclusive child care programmes, outdoor play can be a major challenge. Music interventions facilitate play and involve peers in interaction, and they can also encourage meaningful play on the playground.

Music therapy as a cognitive development intervention

Cognitive intervention is most effective if based upon a child's cognitive strengths and weaknesses and the interrelationships of cognitive development with sensory-motor, language and behavioural growth. Research on learning among all types of children has pointed to the importance of the early years. For children with Fragile X syndrome, these early years are of vital importance for stimulating maximum learning.

Music therapy is based on the activity of playing improvised music in a therapeutic relationship. Clearly the activity of listening, in a structured musical improvisational context, without the lexical demands of language, is a platform for communicational improvement. The building blocks of language, rhythm, articulation and sequencing are musical in nature. Focused listening to another person is also a prerequisite of effective mutual communication, dialogue and social interaction.

Hand and eye coordination, which are dependent on a wider body awareness, appear to be the third vital component in developmental change. Hand movement plays an important role in non-verbal communication and gesture, in the subtle aspects of emotional expression, the acquisition of language and in cognitive development. The integration of cognitive, gestural, emotional and relational abilities is the strength of active music therapy for developmentally challenged children. The activation of hand and eye coordination, as visual-semantic and gestural schema, influences speech-related practical reasoning.

Music and infants

Music soothes, and the existence of the lullaby is presumptive evidence that mothers have always, or nearly always, believed that it can quieten babies. For over a quarter of a century evidence has accumulated that music might improve the physiological responses and growth of premature infants. Premature infants in the intensive care unit are often subjected to levels of environmental noise which cause concern, but the special properties of music may make it beneficial. A general consensus from accumulated research results shows that music is good for premature infants. Both male and female infants in hospital show an improved tolerance for stimulation.

Music therapy is an important intervention that is soothing for the infant. Perhaps as important, music therapy can also encourage parental involvement, support infant development and optimise pre-term neuro-developmental outcomes. Music reduces stress in premature infants.

Music making and music therapy bring about some of the developmental changes necessary to achieving communicative interaction, and this is the basis of social interaction and independence. Listening and performing in the musical relationship, i.e. action and purposeful movement in a relational context, are the building blocks of developmental change. That these factors are pre-verbal, and not lexically dependent, would argue for the importance of music making in the treatment of developmentally delayed infants.

Music therapy reduces anxiety, promotes non-verbal interaction and dialogue, specifically enhances the prosodic elements of communication, encourages sensory integration, manages arousal and provides a platform for cognitive abilities.

We recommend a service which:

- encourages music making through singing and vocalisation between caregivers and babies

- offers specific music therapy interventions for infants and develops musical resources for parents and children

- offers a specific music therapy intervention for individual children diagnosed with Fragile X syndrome

- offers group music therapy for children with developmental delay

- promotes a social and educational setting for parents and care-givers where parents can be informed of new developments in clinical practice, obtain counselling and encourage self-help.

THINGS TO REMEMBER ABOUT THERAPY

First, there is no magic bullet. You will have to bring different interventions together because this is not simply a medical problem, it involves your child's education and his or her psychological social welfare.

Second, try to avoid being a 'photographer'. Photographers develop negatives. You will find any number of professionals who know exactly what your child cannot do. That is how they discover a clinical diagnosis and can make a referral for specialist help. However, you know what your child *can do*. Try to find activities that build upon your child's potentials.

Third, do not overburden your child with too many activities. A long day at school followed by speech therapy and then music therapy can overtax both your child and you. Find an activity where your child can play and simply *be*. Arts and sports activities are great for helping your child simply be him- or herself, particularly in a social setting.

Finally, you will be the coordinator and you have the overview. Make sure you get your own support. Ask for help for you and your child. This help may come from self-help groups, friends and family, or professionals. There no longer needs to be a stigma attached to an intellectually disabled child. There are other people out there and they will be willing to help.

Sensory issues

Occupational and arts therapists with sensory integration knowledge can work with the child and advise parents and carers. Because sensory problems are common, particularly in boys affected by Fragile X, excess stimulation can cause stress, anxiety and problems with concentration and behaviour. Sensory defensiveness influences learning negatively so it is important to find a therapist with skills in this area.

Children may be hypersensitive to sounds, smells and tastes that may be too strong for them. Touch can be too intense and visual stimuli too much to process adequately. However, for some children the opposite may be true: they are hyposensitive and not getting enough stimuli.

Calming techniques reduce anxiety, and improve concentration and learning, which helps prevent inappropriate behaviour and enables the child to adjust to his or her surroundings. Similarly, reducing strong stimuli that cause distress or techniques for preparing children in advance are important.

Gross motor skills, like crawling, walking, running, jumping and throwing balls are important skills for children to learn. Physiotherapy, sensory integration therapy and adapted physical education activities are of help if gross motor problems exist.

Writing, drawing, using a knife and fork and fastening buttons are just a few examples of the many activities that require fine motor skills. Occupational therapists help children improve their fine motor skills by assessing where areas of difficulty are occurring and tailoring activities to improve skills. A therapist can also provide oral and facial activities, to help with mouth sensitivity issues.

Physical activities improve sensory integration skills by giving children practice in using their body in different ways, helping them learn how it relates to their surroundings. Sports activities are important in helping sensory integration, improving motor skills and developing social integration skills.

Chapter 7

TALKING WITH THE FAMILY

Alicia and Daniel visited their paediatrician to talk about their son, Adrian. After a series of previous consultations, and a genetic test, they are ready to hear the result of that genetic test. Adrian is a boy with Fragile X. Their first reaction is one of shock. Their doctor explains to them all the various ramifications of the diagnosis and the next steps forward. However, all the parents can think about is that the problem is hereditary and has been passed on through Alicia. They return home feeling guilty and lost. Rather than tell the rest of the family, they decide to keep it to themselves. As time passes, Alicia and Daniel have difficulty in coping with Adrian. Daniel spends less and less time at home and eventually they separate.

The immediate impact of a diagnosis that a child has a disability is one of shock. Parents feel very much alone. This shock is further compounded by guilt and loss. Such knowledge, while identifying the source of the problem and confirming what we know intuitively, also brings a flood of other feelings. It is those feelings of shock, guilt, fear for the future and then anger that we need to discuss with our families, friends and professionals. Yet, paradoxically, we often do the opposite, keeping such feelings to ourselves. We enter into a state of denial. This is partly because of the stigma attached to disability, partly because of our often clouded understanding of genetics and partly because it's a simple protective mechanism. In the long term, denial can be debilitating.

What we know is that a diagnosis can be overwhelming emotionally and intellectually. First, we may experience a profound sense of loss. We have lost that perfect child we anticipated. In a modern world where everyone has to be effective, productive, perfectly formed and clever, we know our child is going to fail on some of those counts. All the images of people we have known with disabilities come to the fore. There are few positive role models of people with intellectual disabilities, although we know that such children are rewarding and fulfilling for us as parents. Initially, our thoughts may be very bleak indeed. The problem is that no one can tell us exactly how the syndrome will be expressed. That is why we emphasise early intervention, looking for support and talking to other people.

That sense of loss can then lead to a fear for the future. As soon as we know of a diagnosis, we then begin to project that knowledge into the future. How is my child going to fit into school? Will he or she have to go to a special school? Will he or she be able to speak properly? Will he or she be able to make friends and have some sort of independence? By talking to other people who have been in the same situation, we can see how they have coped. Some of our fears can be allayed. We can also see that taking things one step at a time is a necessary strategy.

We refer to this as a loss because we lose an idealised future as parents and our idealised view of what we will be as a family. We also expect that our children will eventually leave home. We speculate on how long we will have to care for them and then what will happen when we too are infirm? In some ways, we have lost a dream and that is painful. Maybe the dream was never stated specifically but we all make plans as parents and have hopes for our futures and those of our children. If we can grasp that our child, although having a disability, is a valuable person, who will cherish us and needs what we have to offer, then we can begin to construct an alternative positive dream for the future.

Second, there is often a feeling of guilt that we may have caused the problem. Given that, for many of us, genetics is an opaque discipline and sometimes a taboo, it is not surprising that our thinking may be confused at first. Heredity happens. We do it all the time when we have children or, as geneticists say, offspring. Passing on our genetic code from one generation to the next is a natural activity. It is not something we do intentionally. Although we may believe choosing a mate is a rational activity, biology plays a primary role. One of the difficulties is that we are so used to thinking about ourselves, and our own decision-making, in terms of personal agency. We forget that we are also a species that passes on its genetic material over generations. To ensure our survival as a species, we need bio-diversity. This is a fact of our material being; we are creatures in the natural world and our cells follow the laws of nature. Nobody is to blame. Nature happens. We are brutally confronted with the limits of what we can do personally.

We are not simply natural beings, and of course we all seek a reason for what has happened. Sometimes people think they are being punished, or they did something wrong during pregnancy, or chose the wrong diet. Some people blame their partners once there have been genetic tests in the wider family. This guilt is a natural reaction to the reality of what has happened. We seek to make sense of the diagnosis and often, when the pain is too much, to lay the blame somewhere. But no one is to blame. We are part of a natural world.

Some people do feel that they are being punished in some way or that God has given them a burden. All we can recommend is talking to people with an intellectually disabled child. We can also turn around that feeling of being burdened to see that maybe we have been chosen for a special task because we have something extra to offer. Children are a blessing. At times when we are dramatically challenged with the realisation that our child will be intellectually disabled, and experiencing all the negative feelings of loss, confusion and disappointment, we ask that question: 'Why me?' All too often this is interpreted negatively because we are experiencing the loss. However, maybe we have to ask the question neutrally and wait for the answer to show itself positively. If it really is a serious question for the religiously or spiritually minded then the answer to 'Why me?' will be 'Because you have something special to offer to your child'.

However, while being confronted with the neutrality of nature, we also have to bring together our personal resources, and those of our family, to do something for our child in the future. Although there is support out there, it will fall to the parents or caregivers to rally that support and coordinate help. We are gradually marshalling professional expertise worldwide, and research is growing each year, but in the end it is the parents who have to pull all those initiatives together for their child. While the problem is biological and initially identified as medical, the consequences for the child's life will be educational, psychological, medical and social. Each agency will have something to offer; bringing those agencies together falls as a task to the parents.

Not knowing is the greatest hindrance initially and that is why we recommend talking to as many people as possible. The national Fragile X associations will have resources and know people in your locality (see the list of web links at the end of this book). Through the confusion of the early days, when it is easy to be overloaded with information, we need people to talk to who can speak clearly with us. One of the problems is that when we are in a state of shock it is difficult to take things in and make sense of all the information that comes to us. That is why it is important that we do not close down and not tell anyone, but instead seek out people who are knowledge-able and give us time.

It is understandable that when families are confronted with such a diagnosis and receive a confirmation of the condition they may feel emotionally overwhelmed by the complexity of the disorder and the implications this has for the family. This is where genetic counsellors are important in advising about the genetics of the condition and im-plications for other family members. Counsellors offer support prior to and during testing, throughout the process of making decisions based on the results of testing, and can offer ongoing follow-up.

We know that families go through stages of feeling stigmatised, estranged and isolated and may exhibit poor self-esteem and self-image. As with any perceived loss, family members will tend to go through a range of feelings including guilt, anger, grief and denial. These feelings will also tend to reappear as the child with Fragile X moves through the different life stages. Support systems need to be identified and encouraged, as there is an ongoing need for monitoring and support.

Women with a family history of Fragile X syndrome need to be offered genetic counselling with informed consent. Female carriers of the pre-mutation must be informed of the possible risk of reduced fertility, which has implications for deciding at what age to try to conceive children, and for the decisions about prenatal or pre-implantational diagnosis.

The whole concept of being a 'carrier' is difficult and can damage our self-identities. However, we all carry genetic material and pass this on as a matter of course. It is only when there are potentially negative outcomes that our awareness is aroused. For women, as we have seen, questions are raised about having biological children and the implications for grandchildren. Affected women really need to discuss this with their genetic counsellor and talk about a positive identity, particularly when they are considered as being 'at risk'.

For men, the discovery of FXTAS means that male pre-mutated carriers must become aware of their potential for developing clinical symptoms. When the diagnosis of Fragile X syndrome is made of a child in a family, then testing of the maternal grandparents is recommended. Often, the grandfather is close to the age for the onset of FXTAS. Again, this means a changed identity that demands coping skills.

The diagnosis of Fragile X has implications for the rest of the family. In general it is possible to approach the family and discuss what the diagnosis implies; although this is supposed to be an advantage, there are occasions where ethical conflicts occur and a family indicates they do not want to inform the rest of the family members. What is important is that we make a shift from the concept of the individual patient, to that of helping a family muster their coping resources. This does not mean making the family 'the patient'. It simply means locating medical understandings within a broader framework of understandings.

Where children less than 18 years old are concerned, discussing a diagnosis of Fragile X in their brother or sister is a delicate matter.

This is where the genetic counsellor really does need to be given a prominent role as he or she will have the basic factual understanding in place. As parents you will bring the emotional understanding of your own child, and this will vary according to his or her age and personality. If you as parents have a positive understanding of what the diagnosis means then it is easier to pass on this positive attitude to your other children. Your children will need to know because if they too are carriers, this will affect their decisions to have children in the future.

CONCLUSION

We have mentioned blame here, in terms of not blaming the child nor the parents for behavioural problems. It is also important to say that because this is a genetic disorder, we do not need to blame ourselves for our genetic make-up, nor our forebearers who have passed on this legacy to us. But, with modern scientific knowledge, we can now know what we are passing on to the next generations.

Over the past few decades, advances in genetics and genomics have changed the possibilities we have to think about health and illness. Genetics has been traditionally associated with pregnancy and birth defects but is now influencing how we think about how we can modify the human being. So we are not solely dealing with biological characteristics but also having to answer complex questions of ethics and social responsibility. While we have an increasingly sophisticated scientific genetic understanding, how that knowledge is transferred into everyday practice is still challenging.

A major problem worldwide is that although Fragile X syndrome is the most common cause of inherited intellectual disability it is often missed as a diagnosis. The reasons behind this failure to recognise or correctly diagnose the condition are mixed. One reason is that not all physicians are geneticists and aware of Fragile X syndrome. With more knowledge of the condition in general practice, amongst paediatricians and neurologists, correct diagnoses will follow. Another reason is that there is a wide variability in how the condition is presented and experienced. As parents, you too can play a significant role in the advancement of knowledge. Knowledge is becoming democratised with the development of the worldwide web. Parents are lobbying their governments and raising awareness. This advocacy leads to an improvement in service from professionals but also makes sure that research serves the people who need it most.

The most important message is that you are not alone, so communicate and connect. Children with an intellectual disability can be rewarding as well as challenging. As a parent you are central to their life. It sometimes appears that after the diagnosis the professionals become the experts, and this may leave a parent 'out in the cold'. As this is often the father, we emphasise the inclusion of both partners in all decision-making.

As parents you will need a lot of support, so ask for it. You will have to look for it at times. Talking does help. As parents, we also need some time to enjoy our lives and as your relationship with your child changes, so will your relationship with your partner and the rest of the family. You will need to make time for your partner and for your other children.

New research is also confirming that parental concerns about their child having a delay in language or motor development are well founded and provide valuable information for the detection of such delay. Therefore, it is important to voice your concerns early to your health care professional. If you have specific concerns it may be helpful to make a video-recording of your child's behaviour and show your doctor or paediatrician.

We often referred to a 'developmental delay' in previous years, rather than 'intellectual disability'. While developmental delay is now considered a negative term, it also kept us alerted to the idea that the family needs to be aware of the delay that may occur in their own relationships. Again, it helps to talk about hopes and dreams and how these change.

None of us is usually successful at predicting the future, so try to keep a short time frame on your expectations. Similarly, no expert can tell you exactly what your child is capable of achieving in the future. It is often our unrealistic expectations that are the basis for our disappointments. Enjoy your child as he or she is.

Start early finding help and learning about disability. You will become the expert for your child and you can use this expertise to help others.

BOX 7.1 SOME TIPS FOR GETTING HELP AND FINDING SUPPORT

Find a doctor you can talk to.

- This may be your child's paediatrician or your family doctor.

- If you do not understand what your doctor is saying, keep on asking questions.

Ask questions.

- Write your questions down beforehand and keep a notebook of questions to ask and answers you have received, particularly when referred to specialist practitioners or a genetic counsellor.

- Do not apologise for asking. It's your child and you need to know – in a language that you can understand.

Ask more questions, find experts.

- Do not be intimidated by experts: it is your child and you have to wake up with him or her and get him or her to bed at night.

You are the expert on your own child.	▪ Parental concerns about language and motor development are considered to be good indicators of developmental delay.
Keep on learning.	▪ Learn more about the syndrome from specialist Fragile X organisations (see the section on web links at the end of this book).
	▪ Read the resources on the web and ask the professionals what they have as reading material or which they can recommend.
Contact your local Fragile X association.	▪ These are excellent sources of support and information.
Contact your local education, social and psychological services.	▪ Check out early intervention services so that you can begin as soon as possible to start a plan for your child.
	▪ Check out the rights that your child has in terms of special education and any related services.
Find a self-help group and join it.	▪ You are not alone and many others have been this way before or are travelling it now. You need them, they need you.

BOX 7.2 SOME BASIC CONSIDERATIONS

Personal
- Your child will be rewarding.
- You have much to offer.
- Talking helps: find someone to talk to.

Parental
- Parents need support – you do the bulk of the work and need to take care of yourselves.
- The parental relationship is absolutely essential, so you need to look after it by making time for each other.
- All relationships change over time.

Familial
- Families change and children grow up. When a child has special needs, those changes can be very demanding.
- Siblings need support too.

Existential
- Try not to predict the future – it happens anyway, though it may not match our expectations.

Educational
- Start interventions early.
- Learn about intellectual disability – you are the expert.

GLOSSARY

Adenine (A)
One of the building blocks of the nucleic acid molecules of *DNA* and *RNA*.

Adrenergic receptor antagonists
The adrenergic receptors are involved in the body's fight-or-flight response; heart rate increases and pupils dilate, energy is mobilised and blood flow diverted from other non-essential organs to skeletal muscle. This can appear as the symptoms of hyperactivity. Pharmaceutical research is developing blockers (antagonists) that help children who are emotionally overwhelmed and reduce their anxiety.

Allele
One form of a pair of *gene* variants located at a specific position on a *chromosome*.

Amino acid
The building blocks from which *proteins* are constructed.

Ataxia
A lack of coordination of muscle movements, especially at the extremities.

Base
Shortened version of nitrogenous base, the building blocks of nucleic acid molecules (A = *adenine*; T = *thymine*; G = *guanine*; C = *cytosine*; U = *uracil*). The nitrogenous bases bond as complementary pairs between opposing strands of *DNA*.

Base pair
Two complementary nucleotide bases in *DNA* (*A* with *T*; *G* with *C*).

Chromosome
A threadlike structure appearing in a cell nucleus consisting of the *genes* necessary for the transmission of hereditary characteristics. In the human species there are 23 pairs of chromosomes (46 in total).

CpG island
A DNA region rich in *CG* (see *Base*) located upstream of approximately 56 per cent of the genes in the human genome.

Cytogenetic analysis
The study and analysis of *chromosomes*, their structure, function and abnormalities.

Cytosine (C)
One of the building blocks of the nucleic acid molecules of *DNA* and *RNA*.

Delection
Loss of a sequence of *DNA* or part of a *chromosome*.

Diploid
A cell with two sets of *chromosomes*, or double the *haploid* number of chromosomes in the germ cell, with one member of each chromosome pair derived from the egg and one from the sperm. The diploid number, 46 in humans, is the normal chromosome complement of an organism's body cells.

DNA (deoxyribonucleic acid)
An extremely long molecule that is the main component of *chromosomes* and is the material that transfers genetic characteristics in all life forms. A nucleic acid consists of two long chains of *nucleotides* twisted together. The genetic information of DNA is encoded in the sequence of the *bases* in the nucleotide strands and this information is transcribed as the strands unwind and replicate.

DNA sequencing
Determination of the order of *nucleotides* in a *DNA* molecule.

Expression
The extent to which the effects of a *gene* are manifested.

Fragile site
A non-staining gap in a *chromosome* or chromatic.

Gamete or Germ cell
A sexual reproductive cell, such as a sperm or an egg, that unites with another cell to form a new organism.

Gene
The unit of inheritance, consisting of a sequence of *DNA* that codes for an *RNA* and/or polypeptide molecule.

Genetic counselling
The provision of genetic information to facilitate informed decision-making.

Genotype
The genetic constitution of an organism.

Guanine (G)
One of the building blocks of the nucleic acid molecules of *DNA* and *RNA*.

Haploid
A single set of unpaired *chromosomes* (especially found in the sperm or the egg).

Locus
The position occupied by a *gene* on a *chromosome* relative to the position of other genes on that chromosome.

Methylation

A chemical process in the body that is used to turn chromosome information off or on. In people with Fragile X syndrome, it is this process of methylation that causes the disease by turning genetic information 'off', sometimes known as 'silencing', where the expression of the gene is silenced.

mGluR5 antagonist

Metabotropic glutamate receptor 5 (mGluR5) is a protein involved in normal brain function and neurotransmission. Some researchers suggest that if the activation of mGluR5 goes unchecked we see the clinical symptoms of Fragile X. mGluR5 antagonists are a major part of pharmaceutical research to help restore normal brain function and alleviate symptoms.

Microsatellite

Numerous short segments of *DNA* that are distributed throughout the genome consisting of repeated sequences of usually two to five *nucleotides*. They are often used in genetics as a marker in identifying important genetic traits.

Mosaic (Mosaicism)

A condition in which tissues of genetically different types occur in the same organism.

mRNA (messenger RNA)

A form of *RNA*, transcribed from a single strand of *DNA*, that carries genetic information that specifies the amino acid sequence for *protein* synthesis.

Mutation

Change in the normal structure or sequence of a *gene* that departs from the parent type.

Nucleotide
The basic structural unit of *DNA* and *RNA* made up of sugar, a phosphate group and a nitrogenous base (*adenine*, *cytosine*, *guanine* and *thymine* or *uracil*).

PCR (polymerase chain reaction)
A technique that enables multiple copies of a *DNA* molecule to be generated by enzymatic amplification of a target *DNA* sequence.

Perseveration
Children with intellectual disabilities, particularly those on the autism spectrum, perseverate. Perseverating means they do certain actions over and over again, such as repeating a phrase, shutting a door, twiddling fingers or objects, lining up toys or spinning objects. It is simply the repetition of a behaviour which seems meaningless to the observer as there is no obvious stimulus.

Phenotype
The clinical outcome of an expressed *gene* or genes, which also refers to the outcome of the interaction of genes with environment.

Pre-mutation
A clinically insignificant change in a *gene* which may predispose it to a subsequent full *mutation* that is significant clinically.

Pre-mutation carrier
Men and women can be carriers of a Fragile X mutation. A carrier is an individual who carries an altered form of a gene which can lead to having a child or offspring in future generations with a genetic disorder.

Protein
A complex organic compound composed of hundreds or thousands of *amino acids*.

Ribose
A pentose sugar occurring as a component of *RNA*.

RNA (ribonucleic acid)
A constituent of cells, consisting of a long, usually single-stranded chain of alternating phosphate and *ribose* units with the bases *adenine*, *guanine*, *cytosine* and uracil bonded to the ribose. The structure and base sequence of RNA are determinants of *protein* synthesis and the transmission of genetic information.

Screening
The identification of persons from a population with a particular disorder or those who might carry a *gene* for such a disorder.

Sex chromosomes
The X and Y *chromosomes* responsible for sex type (XX in women and XY in men).

Southern Blot
A diagnosis technique for detecting *DNA* fragments by hybridisation.

Syndrome
A combination of clinical features, or a group of symptoms, forming a recognisable entity such as a specific disorder, condition or a disease.

Thymine (T)
One of the building blocks of the nucleic acid molecules of *DNA* and *RNA*.

Translation
The process of *protein* synthesis from messenger RNA (see *mRNA*) where the messenger RNA directs the assembly of *amino acids* that makes the protein.

Tremor

An involuntary movement of one or more body parts, most often occurring in the hands. An intentional tremor occurs when grasping as opposed to a tremor at rest.

Uracil

One of the building blocks of the nucleic acid molecules of *DNA* and *RNA*.

FURTHER READING

GENERAL WORKS ON FRAGILE X

Cornish, K., Turk, J. and Hagerman, R. (2008) 'The fragile X continuum: New advances and perspectives.' *Journal of Intellectual Disability Research 6*, 52, 469–82.

de Diego-Otero, Y., Romero-Zerbo, Y., El Bekay, R., Decara-Del Olmo, J. *et al.* (2006) 'Experimental models used in research into genetic disorders that involve intellectual disability.' *Neurologia 42*, 1, 85–92.

De Vries, B.B., Halley, D.J., Oostra, B.A. and Niermeijer, M.F. (1998) 'The fragile X syndrome.' *Journal of Medical Genetics 35*, 579–89.

D'Hulst, C. and Kooy, R.F. (2009) 'Fragile X syndrome: from molecular genetics to therapy.' *Journal of Medical Genetics 46*, 9, 577–84. Review.

Greene, R.W. (1998) *The Explosive Child: Understanding and Parenting Easily Frustrated 'Chronically Inflexible' Children.* New York: HarperCollins.

Hagerman, R. (2002) 'The Physical and Behavioral Phenotype.' In R. Hagerman and P. Hagerman (eds) *Fragile X Syndrome: Diagnosis, Treatment and Research.* Baltimore, MD: Johns Hopkins University Press.

Hagerman, R., Amiri, K. and Cronister, A. (1991) 'Fragile X checklist.' *American Journal of Medical Genetics 38*, 283–7.

McConkie-Rosell, A., Finucane, B., Cronister, A., Abrams, L. *et al.* (2005) 'Genetic counseling for Fragile X Syndrome: Update recommendations of the National Society of Genetic Counsellors.' *Journal of Genetic Counseling 14*, 4, 249–70.

Medved, M.I. and Brockmeier, J. (2004) 'Making sense of traumatic experiences: Telling your life with Fragile X Syndrome.' *Qualitative Health Research 14*, 6, 741–59.

Nolin, S.L., Lewis, F.A., Ye, L.L., Houck, G.E. *et al.* (1996) 'Familial transmission of the FMR1 GCC repeat.' *American Journal of Human Genetics 59*, 1252–61.

Oostra, B.A. and Chiurazzi, P. (2001) 'The fragile X gene and its function.' *Clinical Genetics 60*, 399–408.

Roberts, J., Boccia, M.L., Bailey, D.B. Jr., Hatton, D.D. and Skinner, M. (2001) 'Cardiovascular indices of physiological arousal in boys with Fragile X syndrome.' *Developmental Psychobiology 39*, 2, 107–23.

Rousseau, F., Heitz, D., Tarleton, J., MacPherson, J. *et al.* (1994) 'A multicenter study on genotype-phenotype correlations in the fragile X syndrome, using direct diagnosis with probe StB12.3: The first 2,253 cases.' *American Journal of Human Genetics 55*, 225–37.

Scharfenaker, S., O'Connor, R., Stackhouse, T., Braden, M. *et al.* (2002) 'An Integrated Approach to Intervention.' In R. Hagerman and P. Hagerman (eds) *Fragile X Syndrome: Diagnosis, Treatment and Research.* Baltimore, MD: John Hopkins University Press.

Visootsak, J., Wareen, S.T., Anido, A. and Gram, J.M. Jr. (2005) 'Fragile X syndrome: An update and review for the primary paediatrician.' *Clinical Pediatrics 44*, 371–81.

PRE-MUTATION DISORDERS IN ADULTS: FRAGILE X-ASSOCIATED TREMOR/ATAXIA SYNDROME AND PREMATURE OVARIAN INSUFFICIENCY

Allingham-Hawkins, D.J., Babul-Hirji, R., Chitayat, D., Holden, J.J. *et al.* (1999) 'Fragile X premutation is a significant risk factor for premature ovarian failure: The International Collaborative POF in Fragile X study – preliminary data.' *American Journal of Medical Genetics 83*, 322–5.

Baba, Y. and Uitti, R.J. (2005) 'Fragile X-associated tremor/ataxia syndrome and movements disorders.' *Current Opinion in Neurology 18*, 4, 393–8.

Bretherick, K.L., Fluker, M.R. and Robinson, W.P. (2005) 'FMR1 repeat sizes in the gray zone and high end of the normal range are associated with premature ovarian failure.' *Journal of Human Genetics 117*, 4, 376–82.

Fernández, I., López, B., Alonso, M.J., Telleria, J.J. *et al.* (2005) 'Study of the phenotype of unrelated patients (males and females) with premutation and intermediate alleles of FMR1.' *Journal of Human Genetics 13*, 135.

Greco, C.M., Hagerman, R.J., Tassone, F., Chudley, A.E. *et al.* (2002) 'Neuronal intranuclear inclusions in a new cerebellar tremor/ataxia syndrome among fragile X carriers.' *Brain 125*, 1760–71.

Hagerman, P. and Hagerman, R. (2004) 'The Fragile-X premutation: A maturing perspective.' *American Journal of Human Genetics 74*, 805–16.

Hagerman, P. and Hagerman, R. (2004) 'Fragile X-associated tremor/ataxia syndrome (FXTAS)'. *Mental Retardation and Developmental Disabilities Research Reviews 10*, 25–30.

Hagerman, R., Hall, D., Coffey, S., Leehey, M. *et al.* (2008) 'Treatment of fragile X-associated tremor ataxia syndrome (FXTAS) and related neurological problems.' *Clinical Interventions in Aging 3*, 2, 251–62.

Hall, D.A., Howard, K., Hagerman, R. and Leehey, M.A. (2009) 'Parkinsonism in FMR1 premutation carriers may be indistinguishable from Parkinson disease.' *Parkinsonism and Related Disorders 15*, 2, 156–9.

Leehey, M.A., Munhoz, R.P., Lang, A.E., Brunberg, J.A. *et al.* (2003) 'The fragile X premutation presenting as essential tremor.' *Archives of Neurology 60*, 117–21.

Murray, A., Ennis, S., MacSwiney, F., Webb, J. and Morton, N.E. (2000) 'Reproductive and menstrual history of females with fragile X expansions.' *European Journal of Human Genetics 8*, 247–52.

Tejada, M.I., Gracia-Alegria, A., Bilbao, C., Martines-Bouzas, E. *et al.* (2008) 'Analysis of the molecular parameters which could predict the risk of manifesting Premature Ovarian Failure (POF) in female permutation carriers of Fragile X Syndrome.' *Menopause 15,* 5, 945–9.

AUTISM AND ATTENTION DEFICIT HYPERACTIVITY DISORDER

Barkley, R.A. (1995) *Taking Charge of ADHD: A Complete, Authoritative Guide for Parents.* New York: Guilford Press.

Belmonte, M.K. and Bourgeron, T. (2006) 'Fragile X syndrome and autism at the intersection of genetic and neural networks.' *Nature Neuroscience 9*, 10, 1221–5.

Clifford, S., Dissanayake, C., Bui, Q.M., Huggins, R., Taylor, A.K. *et al.* (2007) 'Autism spectrum phenotype in males and females with fragile X full mutation and premutation.' *Journal of Autism and Developmental Disorders 37*, 738–47.

Lathe, R. (2009) 'Fragile X and autism.' *Autism 13*, 2, 194–7.

Macedoni-Luksic, M., Greiss-Hess, L., Rogers, S.J., Gosar, D., Lemons-Chitwood, K. and Hagerman, R. (2009) 'Imitation in fragile X syndrome: Implications for autism.' *Autism 13*, 6, 599–611.

Marco, E.J. and Skuse, D.H. (2006) 'Autism: Lessons from the X chromosome.' *Social Cognitive and Affective Neuroscience 1*, 3, 183–93.

Rogers, S.J., Wehner, D.E. and Hagerman, R. (2001) 'The behavioral phenotype in Fragile X: Symptoms of autism in very young children with Fragile X syndrome, idiopathic autism, and other developmental disorders.' *Journal of Developmental and Behavioral Pediatrics 22*, 6, 409–17.

SCREENING AND TESTING

Fernández, I., Telleria, J.J., Blanco, A., Alonso, M.J. *et al.* (2001) 'Effectiveness of a clinical test in the preselection of children with suspected fragile X syndrome.' *Anales de Pediatría 54*, 4, 227–31.

Fernández-Carvajal, I., Lopez Posadas, B., Pan, R., Raske, C. *et al.* (2009) 'Expansion of an FMR1 grey-zone allele to a full mutation in two generations.' *Journal of Molecular Diagnosis 11*, 4, 306–10.

Fernandez-Carvajal, I., Walichiewicz, P., Xiaosen, X., Pan, R. *et al.* (2009) 'Screening for expanded alleles of the FMR1 gene in blood spots from newborn males in a Spanish population.' *Journal of Molecular Diagnosis 11,* 4, 324–9.

Gedeon, A.K., Baker, E., Robinson, H., Partington, M.W. *et al.* (1992) 'Fragile X syndrome without CCG amplification has an FMR1 deletion.' *Nature Genetics 1*, 341–4.

Govaerts, L., Smit, A., Saris, J., Vanderwerf, F. *et al.* (2007) 'Exceptional good cognitive and phenotypic profile in a male carrying a mosaic mutation in the FMR1 gene.' *Clinical Genetics 72*, 138–44.

Jacquemont, S., Farzin, F., Hall, D., Leehey, M. *et al.* (2004) 'Aging in individuals with the FMR1 mutation.' *American Journal of Mental Retardation 109*, 154–64.

Lopez, B., Alonso, M., Blanco, A., Aldridge, D. and Fernandez-Carvajal, I. (2010) 'Evaluation of FMR1 grey alleles stability and its risk of expansion upon transmission.' *Molecular Syndromology 1*, 154.

McConkie-Rosell, A., Lachiewicz, A.M., Spiridigliozzi, G.A., Tarleton, J. *et al.* (1993) 'Evidence that methylation of the FMR-1 locus is responsible for variable phenotypic expression of the fragile X syndrome.' *American Journal of Human Genetics 53*, 800–809.

Pembrey, M.E., Barnicoat, A.J., Carmichael, B., Bobrow, M. and Turner, G. (2001) 'An assessment of screening strategies for fragile X syndrome in the UK.' *Health Technology Assessment 5*, 7, 1–95.

Sherman, S., Pletcher, B.A. and Driscoll, D.A. (2005) 'Fragile X syndrome: Diagnostic and carrier testing.' *Genetics in Medicine 7*, 8, 584–7.

Tassone, F., Pan, R., Amiri, K., Taylor, A.K. and Hagerman, P.J. (2008) 'A rapid polymerase chain reaction-based screening method for identification of all expanded alleles of the fragile X (FMR1) gene in newborn and high-risk populations.' *Journal of Molecular Diagnostics 10*, 1, 43–9.

Taylor, A.K. (1994) 'Fragile X DNA testing: A guide for physicians and families.' In Fragile X Foundation Educational files. Volume 2. Available at www.fragilex.org/html/diagnosis.htm, accessed on 10 October 2010.

Verkerk, A.J.M., Pieretti, M., Sutcliffe, J.S., Fu, Y. *et al.* (1991) 'Identification of a gene (FMR-1) containing a CGG repeat coincident with a breakpoint cluster region exhibiting length variation in fragile X syndrome.' *Cell 65*, 905–14.

Yu, S., Pritchard, M., Kremer, E., Lynch, M. *et al.* (1991) 'Fragile X genotype characterized by an unstable region of DNA.' *Science 252*, 1179–81.

MUSIC THERAPY AS SPECIFIC INTERVENTIONS

Aldridge, D. (1996) *Music Therapy Research and Practice: From Out of the Silence.* London: Jessica Kingsley Publishers.

Aldridge, D., Gustorff, D. and Neugebauer, L. (1995) 'A pilot study of music therapy in the treatment of children with developmental delay.' *Complementary Therapies in Medicine 3*, 197–205.

Kern, P. and Aldridge, D. (2006) 'Using embedded music therapy interventions to support outdoor play of young children with autism in an inclusive community-based child care program.' *Journal of Music Therapy 43*, 4, 270–94.

Kern, P., Wakeford, L. and Aldridge, D. (2007) 'Improving the performance of a young child with autism during self-care tasks using embedded song interventions: A case study.' *Music Therapy Perspectives 25*, 1, 43–51.

Kern, P., Wolery, M. and Aldridge, D. (2006) 'Use of songs to promote independence in morning greeting routines for young children with autism.' *Journal of Autism and Developmental Disorders 37*, 7, 1264–71.

SOCIAL SKILLS

Reichow, B. and Volkmar, F. (2010) 'Social skills interventions for individuals with autism: Evaluation for evidence-based practices within a best evidence synthesis framework.' *Journal of Autism and Developmental Disorders 40*, 149–66.

FRAGILE X WEB LINKS

The following are general umbrella websites listing Fragile X societies worldwide:

www.fragilex.org/html/international.htm

www.fragilex.org.uk/FragileX/FragileXGroupsOverseas/tabid/67/Default.aspx

AUSTRALIA

Fragile X Alliance Inc.
www.fragilex.com.au

Fragile X Association of Australia
www.fragilex.org.au

CANADA

Fragile X Research Foundation of Canada
www.fragilexcanada.ca

GERMANY

Interessengemeinschaft Fragiles-X e.V.
www.frax.de

INDIA

Fragile X Society – India
www.fragilex.org/html/india.htm

IRELAND

Irish Fragile X Society
www.fragilex-ireland.org

NEW ZEALAND

Fragile X Trust New Zealand
www.fragilex.org.nz/home

SPAIN

Federación Española Síndrome X Frágil
www.nova.es/xfragil

USA

FRAXA Research Foundation
A non-profit organisation run by parents and an excellent source of information.
www.fraxa.org

The National Fragile X Foundation
www.fragilex.org/html/home.shtml

Especially for Fragile X-associated tremor/ataxia syndrome (FXTAS)
www.fxtas.org

UK

The Fragile X Society
www.fragilex.org.uk

Your Genes Your Health
An informative site about genes and health called Your Genes Your
Health has a special section related to Fragile X:
www.yourgenesyourhealth.org/index.htm

www.yourgenesyourhealth.org/fragx/whatisit.htm

For children

Kids' Health
A special website for children called Kids' Health has a special page
for learning disabilities. This is part of the Children, Youth and
Women's Health Service in South Australia.
www.cyh.com/HealthTopics/HealthTopicDetailsKids.
aspx?p=335&np=285&id=1549

The site also covers what rights and responsibilities are with a further
range of interesting topics.
www.cyh.com/HealthTopics/HealthTopicDetailsKids.
aspx?p=335&np=287&id=1712#1

INDEX